Perspectives in Nursing Management and Care for Older Adults

Series Editors

Julie Santy-Tomlinson
School of Health Sciences
University of Manchester
Manchester, UK

Paolo Falaschi
Sant'Andrea Hospital
Sapienza University of Rome
Rome, Italy

Karen Hertz
University Hospitals of North Midlands
Royal Stoke University Hospital
Stoke-on-Trent, Staffordshire, UK

W0043507

The aim of this book series is to provide a comprehensive guide to nursing management and care for older adults, addressing specific problems in nursing and allied health professions. It provides a unique resource for nurses, enabling them to provide high-quality care for older adults in all care settings. The respective volumes are designed to provide practitioners with highly accessible information on evidence-based management and care for older adults, with a focus on practical guidance and advice.

Though demographic trends in developed countries are sometimes assumed to be limited to said countries, it is clear that similar issues are now affecting rapidly developing countries in Asia and South America. As such, the series will not only benefit nurses working in Europe, North America, Australasia and many developed countries, but also elsewhere. Offering seminal texts for nurses working with older adults in both inpatient and outpatient settings, it will especially support them during the first five years after nurse registration, as they move towards specialist and advanced practice. The series will also be of value to student nurses, employing a highly accessible style suitable for a broader readership.

More information about this series at http://www.springer.com/series/15860

Sarah Ryan
Editor

Nursing Older People with Arthritis and other Rheumatological Conditions

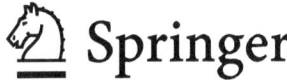 Springer

Editor
Sarah Ryan
Midlands Partnership NHS Foundation Trust
Haywood Hospital
Stoke-On-Trent
Staffordshire
UK

ISSN 2522-8838   ISSN 2522-8846   (electronic)
Perspectives in Nursing Management and Care for Older Adults
ISBN 978-3-030-18011-9   ISBN 978-3-030-18012-6   (eBook)
https://doi.org/10.1007/978-3-030-18012-6

This Springer imprint is published by the registered company Springer Nature Switzerland AG
The registered company address is: Gewerbestrasse 11, 6330 Cham, Switzerland

Foreword

I was delighted to be asked by Professor Sarah Ryan to write the foreword for this important reference book for health professionals, in different settings, who are managing the older adult with one or more of the musculoskeletal diseases (MSDs) included within its scope.

I have lived with severe refractory inflammatory polyarthritis (diagnosed originally as rheumatoid arthritis) for nearly 40 years and have understood, rather better than I would like, the complexities of managing the impact of long-term chronic disease and its comorbidities and complications. People diagnosed many years ago, like myself, have seen the treatment and care of rheumatological disease revolutionised by the advent of new therapies (biologics, biosimilars and the targeted synthetic drugs) and the way in which these diseases are now treated, using aggressive treatments, to target strategies that have transformed care and patients' lives. These advances mean that patients like me, with huge amounts of irreversible damage, many surgeries under our belt and negative impacts of long-term steroid use, are hopefully a thing of the past. With patients who are diagnosed today having the chance of leading a more normal life.

However, there remain many thousands of older people who need the support and understanding of health professionals in different settings, and this book will be enormously beneficial in assessing and treating such patients.

From the patient perspective, there are a number of areas I would like to highlight which I hope will be helpful when assessing someone with RA or other musculoskeletal disease. It's important to take a holistic view of your patient and consider the biopsychosocial aspects of their condition rather than the purely clinical, medical and physical components of disease. Anxiety and depression are common comorbidities, and in all the social surveys and reports NRAS has done over many years, they come out top or near the top of a very long list of comorbidities experienced by people with RA. People with inflammatory arthritis are also at much greater risk of cardiovascular disease (CVD), and in fact, many die earlier than they should due to CVD. Osteoporosis and osteopenia are also common in the older adult with MSDs due to poor mobility and function, leading to a lack of physical activity and exercise.

Social aspects of the person's circumstances also play a major part in anxiety, low mood and depression, such as being isolated from family, having few friends to depend upon for support and being unable to get out independently. Financial circumstances have a significant impact too. Having the ability to heat your home sufficiently, afford help in the house and garden if you are on your own and order in a takeaway meal if you are in too much pain to cook for yourself all make a massive difference to being able to cope and look after yourself independently. Lack of independence takes away dignity and increases anxiety and worry.

When hospitalised for elective surgery, I have frequently found that the nursing staff do not appreciate just how disabled people with RA and other MSDs can be. Disability is not always visible. Being told you need to get out of bed after a joint replacement and sit in a chair can be impossible without substantial help and lifting which is not encouraged or even allowed today, and these seemingly small incidents can cause enormous distress for the patient. Post-operative rehabilitation is another nightmare scenario for so many older patients, particularly those living alone. Having had four major operations on my feet and ankles, our helpline usually ask me to speak to people about to undergo similar surgery, and the major concerns are not so much about the operation itself but how they are going to manage afterwards. No-one really spends time to go into the detail of what the individual is going to need to arrange and put in place. I recall speaking at length to a 72-year-old lady recently who was in a complete state of panic about how she would be able to cope not being able to weight bear for 10–12 weeks. No-one from her healthcare team either in primary or secondary care (least of all the surgeon) was addressing her fears and worries.

Primary care nurses I have found, whilst expert at doing our regular monitoring and generally supportive, have had little training in the management of MSDs, particularly inflammatory autoimmune conditions, and so I think this book will be very helpful in primary care settings and for district health nurses who are visiting elderly people at home. It's easy with a disease like RA to slip quietly into disability without anyone really noticing. The slide can be so gradual that even the person themselves may not realise immediately that something they could do 6 months ago can no longer be achieved. Also, if you are not receiving holistic annual reviews (in line with NICE guidelines and quality standards) where comorbidities including emotional and mental health are being measured, you may be unaware that you have developed hypertension or have become prediabetic, for example. It's therefore important for district and health visitors to be aware of potential comorbidities to look out for when seeing older people with MSDs in their homes.

Finally, I would like to say a few words about the importance for all health professionals treating people with long-term chronic musculoskeletal disease to be aware of the patient organisations like NRAS, who specialise in the diseases we are concerned with here. We spend a great deal of time, resource and money supporting not only the patients we serve but also the health professionals who treat them. We have a very wide range of resources and services that provide fantastic support, educational, informational, practical and emotional, which can transform the way in which people cope with their disease day to day, and knowing where to refer your patients for this valuable help is critical. There are many patient organisations across Europe and in the United States, Canada, Australia and elsewhere that provide information, education and support for patients with a broad range of musculoskel-etal diseases. My impression is that patient organisations are less prevalent and well-established in Africa and the Indian sub-continent, as we do get people from these areas using NRAS resources. The resources available from patient organisa-tions vary from country to country, but it is definitely worthwhile seeking out your local country patient organisation to find out what resources they have and how they can support patients and health professionals.

I am sure that this book will be of enormous value to health professionals work-ing with patients who live with musculoskeletal disease.

Ailsa Bosworth, MBE
National Patient Champion
National Rheumatoid Arthritis Society (NRAS)
Maidenhead, UK

Nursing Older People with Arthritis and Other Rheumatological Conditions

As the number of older people continues to increase worldwide, there has been a growth in the incidence of arthritis and other rheumatological conditions. Older people living with arthritis tend to have at least one other long-term condition and consequently often require a greater number of medications. Ageing causes certain physiological changes to the body including an increase in body fat, reduced muscle mass, changes in bone density and alterations to anatomical structures including the feet. Such changes can have a negative effect on function and can increase the risk of falls. Along with physical changes, the mood of older people can also be affected. Depression is common in people over the age of 65 years. Triggers for an episode of depression in the older person include bereavement, loneliness and isolation. Older people are often reluctant to seek help for depression, and physical symptoms may be reported rather than any change in emotional wellbeing. Depression can reduce the effectiveness of treatment, and the physiological changes associated with ageing can alter drug absorption, metabolism and excretion, increasing the risk of drug toxicity. Not surprising when considering the numerous physical and psychological challenges of providing care for the older adult, a biopsychosocial, person-centred approach to care is advocated.

This is the first nursing textbook to provide a comprehensive and practical overview of the assessment and management of the older adult with arthritis and other rheumatological conditions. The first five chapters introduce the reader to rheumatological conditions commonly seen in older adults. Osteoarthritis (OA) is a common chronic global health condition and a leading cause of pain and disability in older adults. An estimated 10%–15% of all adults over the age of 60 years have some degree of OA. Polymyalgia rheumatica (PMR) is the commonest inflammatory disease in older people and can prove challenging for the clinician to manage, whilst rheumatoid arthritis (RA) and gout (two other inflammatory conditions) also have a substantial global burden. Osteoporosis is the commonest type of bone disease and the primary reason for a broken bone in the older person. Managing any chronic arthritis condition can be challenging for the older person, and the individual will often require guidance from a health professional to become more confident in taking care of their health.

All of the rheumatological conditions in the older person can impact on physical, psychological and social function, which increases the need for nurses and other health professionals to take a holistic comprehensive assessment to identify the severity and impact of the condition as well as to elicit patient priorities and concerns. Management involves the combination of pharmacological and non-pharmacological interventions with the aim of optimising function at all levels. The impact of illness is usually felt most strongly when it affects a person's ability to engage in their day-to-day activities and limits social participation.

Educating patients on their condition and the management of symptoms including pain, fatigue and low mood and optimising physical function are key treatment targets identified by patients and healthcare professionals alike. Consequently, there are dedicated chapters on pain and fatigue management, the psychological and social aspects of care and optimising function. A dedicated chapter on self- management provides the reader with a range of interventions to use in practice, including action planning, goal setting, patient activation, motivational interviewing and health coaching.

Foot care can often be neglected in arthritis management, yet it is essential to aid mobility and optimise function. The chapter on the foot focuses on the need for assessment, recognition and early treatment of foot problems. Common problems such as nail infections can have serious consequences in autoimmune conditions like rheumatoid arthritis. As the older person will often have comorbidities and will be taking polypharmacy, a knowledge on drug treatment (and the potential for interactions) to manage symptoms and treat the underlying cause of the rheumatological condition is essential. The chapter on drug therapy focuses on the four main classifications of drugs including analgesia, nonsteroidal anti-inflammatory drugs, disease-modifying antirheumatic drugs and biologic treatments.

This book provides an introductory text to the needs of older people with arthritis and other rheumatological conditions. The text is aimed at nurses either new to the speciality of rheumatology, student nurses or nurses who encounter people with rheumatological condition in different healthcare settings. It will provide an opportunity for all nurses to refresh their learning on specific rheumatological conditions, such as OA and PMR, so that when the person is being cared for in a different setting, their other care needs can also be addressed. For example, people with a rheumatologic condition often live with comorbidities including cardiovascular problems and may require joint replacement at some time. The foreword to this book is written by the then-CEO of the National Rheumatoid Arthritis Society (NRAS), Ailsa Bosworth, who describes eloquently what can occur following surgery if the nurse and other health professionals lack knowledge and awareness of the patients' other conditions.

This book provides practical, evidence-based advice on how to address the care needs of older adults with arthritis. All chapter authors are experts working within rheumatology practice, education or research, based in the United Kingdom and Europe. Although the text is primarily aimed at nurses, the content will be relevant to other allied health professionals providing care to older adults with arthritis. Although the focus of this book is on the care needs of the older person with arthritis, many of the principles of care contained within the chapters are transferable to all age groups. The text can also be used for revalidation with each chapter having a range of self-assessment activities that will enable the reader to implement their learning into practice.

Stoke-On-Trent, Staffordshire, UK   Sarah Ryan

Contents

Part I

Arthritis and Other Rheumatological Conditions

Osteoarthritis

1

Gail Parsons and Dottie Roberts

1.1 Learning Outcomes

At the end of this chapter, the nurse will be able to:

1. Describe the aetiology of OA
2. Identify personal-level and joint-level risk factors for OA
3. Explain the signs and symptoms of OA
4. Describe the assessment and diagnosis of an individual with OA
5. Identify the investigations used to diagnose OA
6. Describe the management of an individual with OA, to include conservative and surgical options

1.2 Introduction

OA is one of the most common chronic health conditions and a leading cause of pain and disability among adults (Allen and Golightly 2015). In a systematic review conducted to estimate the global burden of OA, hip and knee arthritis was identified as the 11th leading cause of disability worldwide (Cross et al. 2014). An estimated 250 million people worldwide have knee OA; the knee is the most commonly affected joint, followed by the hand and the hip (O'Neill et al. 2018). The foot and spine are also often affected, although any joint can develop OA.

G. Parsons (✉)
The Dudley Group NHS Foundation Trust, Russells Hall Hospital, Dudley, UK
e-mail: gail.parsons1@nhs.net

D. Roberts
Orthopaedic Nurses Certification Board, Chicago, IL, USA

© Springer Nature Switzerland AG 2020
S. Ryan (ed.), *Nursing Older People with Arthritis and other Rheumatological Conditions*, Perspectives in Nursing Management and Care for Older Adults, https://doi.org/10.1007/978-3-030-18012-6_1

Mechanisms underlying the incidence and progression of OA are not well understood, although research continues into disease genesis. Some modifiable and preventable risk factors have been identified (including obesity) (Cross et al. 2014). The emphasis in health care has been directed at decreasing the impact of the risk factors through patient education for self-management of OA, including providing advice on pain management and limitation of physical disability (Ickinger and Tikly 2014). The only definitive treatment for end-stage OA has been total joint replacement (van der Woude et al. 2016).

To provide effective patient care, nurses need to understand the multifactorial nature of OA and its impact on quality of life.

1.3 Defining Osteoarthritis

OA was previously considered a normal effect of ageing. The deterioration of articular cartilage was assumed to be a 'wear and tear' condition. However, it is now understood to be a complex, multifactorial chronic disease of synovial joints with both modifiable and non-modifiable risk factors (Bortoluzzi et al. 2018). Although loss of articular cartilage remains the hallmark pathological feature of OA, OA is now known to involve the entire joint. Changes occur not only in the bone but also in surrounding soft tissues, including the synovium, menisci and ligaments (O'Neill et al. 2018). These structures can shrink, contributing to a loss of range of motion.

Radiographic evidence for OA includes the presence of osteophytes (bony growth), cysts and sclerosis (abnormal hardening of body tissue), as well as loss of joint space. Clinical OA is defined by history and examination. Radiographic evidence is not always linked to strong clinical symptoms. For example, only 40% of patients with moderate radiographic evidence and 60% of those with severe radiographic evidence of knee OA have symptoms (Palazzo et al. 2016). Diagnosis has, thus, developed to consider both structural change and patient symptoms.

1.4 Risk Factors for Osteoarthritis

Risk factors for OA are divided into person-level factors and joint-level factors (Allen and Golightly 2015; Palazzo et al. 2016). Major risk factors in each category are identified below.

1.4.1 Person-Level Risk Factors

Age is the main risk factor for the development of OA. Prevalence of the disease increases with age, peaking at ages 55–64 years (Bortoluzzi et al. 2018; Palazzo et al. 2016). The effect of ageing has been suggested to include the ageing of chondrocytes with associated blocking of cell production. Increased oxidative stress with an associated increase in free fatty acids and hyperglycaemia are also believed to promote the destruction of cartilage (Bortoluzzi et al. 2018). Ageing is also believed to be linked to systemic inflammation that may contribute to the development of OA. Researchers have found an increase with age in blood levels of C-reactive protein, interleukin (IL) 6 and tumour necrosis factor alpha (Greene and Loeser 2015). The presence of these inflammatory markers has been associated with chronic diseases of ageing.

Gender has been identified as another risk factor for OA. Hip, knee and hand OA occur more often in women than in men. Because the incidence increases around the menopause, the role of hormones in the development of OA has been considered. However, evidence to support a hormonal element is conflicting (Palazzo et al. 2016). The difference between men and women in the occurrence of OA could be simply explained by factors such as bone loss or lack of muscle strength (Palazzo et al. 2016).

Obesity, which has been defined as a body mass index (BMI) greater than 30 kg/mm^2, has been associated strongly with knee OA in particular. For every 5 kg/m^2 increase in BMI, the risk of knee OA has been shown to increase by 35% (Palazzo et al. 2016). This association between BMI and development of knee OA is stronger in women than in men. A loss in weight of 5 kg decreases the risk of developing knee OA by 50% (Palazzo et al. 2016). The related occurrence of metabolic syndrome (obesity, hypertension, hyperglycaemia, insulin resistance and dyslipidaemia) has also been suggested as a risk factor for the development of OA (Bortoluzzi et al. 2018).

1.4.2 Joint-Level Risk Factors

Joint injury can contribute to the development of OA. For example, the knee is one of the most frequently injured joints. Rupture of the anterior cruciate ligament can contribute to early development of OA, as can meniscal damage (Palazzo et al. 2016). Joint damage can also occur from haemophilia. The large number of blood vessels in the synovium can bleed into the joint of a person with haemophilia, injuring cartilage in a vicious cycle that worsens the damage with each occurrence of bleeding (Canadian Hemophilia Society).

Repetitive joint use is also a risk factor for OA. Knee OA has been diagnosed more often in people with occupations that require squatting and kneeling. Hip OA has been associated with prolonged lifting and standing, and hand OA occurs more frequently in people with occupations requiring repetitive small joint use (e.g. computer use) (Palazzo et al. 2016). In addition to vocation, participation in sport has been associated with the development of OA through repetitive, high-intensity or high-impact activity that places a stress on the joints (Palazzo et al. 2016). It is unclear, however, if participation in sport alone increases risk or if the risk is due to sometimes undiagnosed micro-injury.

Abnormal alignment of the joint has been associated with progression of OA. For example, a varus or valgus deformity can place more stress on the knee compartment under greatest compressive stress. This has been shown to increase progression of medial or lateral compartment OA, but the association with disease onset is not clear (Palazzo et al. 2016). In addition, patients with foot or ankle OA have an increased risk of developing knee OA. Foot and ankle problems are common in middle-aged to older adults. Researchers suggest that there also may be a shared biomechanical cause for both foot and ankle problems and knee OA (e.g. pronated foot or the use of inappropriate footwear) (Paterson et al. 2017).

1.5   Impact of Osteoarthritis

OA has been recognised as a major contributor to functional impairment and loss of independence (Zambon et al. 2016). The effect of OA on the ability to perform basic or instrumental activities of daily living has been well-documented. However, other effects of OA are becoming better appreciated and understood. For example, persistent pain as one hallmark of the disease has also been associated with psychological factors such as anxiety and depression, which can affect functional activities. Individual differences have also been recognised in the perception and impact of pain. These variables should be included in a multimodal approach to OA management.

In addition to the personal impact, OA has clear societal and economic consequences. In particular, the pain and physical disability associated with knee OA have contributed to an early exit from work for many people. Researchers have suggested that these indirect costs are likely to exceed other costs of OA treatment (e.g. medications) (Laires et al. 2018).

1.6   Diagnosis

Diagnosis is determined by initially taking a history from the individual who may present at the general practitioner surgery. Joint pain that increases with activity is a key feature of the patient's history (Ickinger and Tikly 2014). It is often the main problem that prompts the patient to seek medical care.

Self-reported assessment tools or professional completed tools may be used as part of the process of assessment and diagnosis (Dawson et al. 1998). Disease-specific Western Ontario and McMaster Osteoarthritis Index (WOMAC) for assessment of hip and knee joint symptoms and Oxford hip or knee score can be used to assist the assessment process.

OA may affect one or several joints including hip, knee, shoulder, spine, ankle and hands.

Specific questions to assist the clinical history taking process are outlined in Fig. 1.1.

Question	Patient response	Practitioner evaluation
What is the reason for your visit today?	I have pain in my joint(s)	Chief complaint should be determined to focus on diagnosis
Please describe your pain?	Dull and throbbing all the time with occasional sharp pain	Type and frequency will aid in diagnosis
How long have you had the pain?	Several months with some days not as bad as others	Onset of symptoms is important
Does the pain vary from day to day?	Yes, dependent on how much I walk or how active I try to be	Exacerbations of osteoarthritis may occur
Is the pain progressively worsening over time?	Yes, getting worse over time	Pain score 0–3 may assist in assessment
Do you experience disturbed sleep due to the pain?	Sometimes, when I try to turn over in bed	Movement and pressure on a joint, e.g. knee or shoulder can disturb sleep if severe
Are you taking any pain relief?	I have tried pain killers – sometimes they help to ease the pain	Non-operative treatment advised initially
Is there any activity that makes the pain worse?	When I put my weight on the joint, when I stand in one position for a long time, when I walk on uneven ground or walk up/down a hill	Weight bearing, twisting and kneeling (knee or hip OA) may increase severity of pain
Are there any activities of daily living you are not able to do due to your painful joint?	Tie my shoelaces, put on my socks/stockings, do my shopping, get in/out of my car	Severe OA of a joint will restrict movement and reduce function contributing to difficulty/inability to carry out specific activities

Fig. 1.1 Questions that can be used when taking a clinical history

1.7 Signs and Symptoms

Symptoms of OA include joint pain, often on movement or weight bearing, which is the most commonly reported symptom (Artese and Grubbs 2017). Loss of joint function, localised swelling, joint stiffness, localised heat around the joint, instability due to muscle weakness and sleep disturbance may also be present. Early morning stiffness of less than 30 minutes, short-term stiffness after resting referred to as 'gelling' and activity-related joint pain are all clinical features of OA. Nodes (Artese and Grubbs 2017) which resemble pea-like structures can be found on the finger joints, and these are referred to as Heberden's nodes (distal interphalangeal joints) and Bouchard nodes (proximal interphalangeal joints). The psychological impact on the individual may include clinical depression, poor motivation and loss of body image (Lin 2008) along with generalised decline in the individual's quality of life (Arthritis Research UK 2018; Rosemann et al. 2008).

1.8 Investigations to Assist in the Diagnosis and Management of OA

1.8.1 X-Rays

Although the diagnosis of OA does not require radiological evidence, radiography (X-ray) can be helpful to assess the joint space, alignment and degree of deformity to determine whether surgery is required. X-ray can also be helpful in cases of diagnosis uncertainty (Fig. 1.2). Osteophyte formation (bony spur formation) may be observed at the articular surface along with bone cyst formation in severe or advanced OA (Hayashi et al. 2016).

Various views may be requested to assess all aspects of the joint and specific views of specific joints, for example, sky line view of patella of the knee to assess for OA when the joint is in flexion of around 30°.

Specific weight-bearing images of the hip or knee joint can determine joint space loss, evidence of osteophyte formation and valgus or varus deformity of the knee joint.

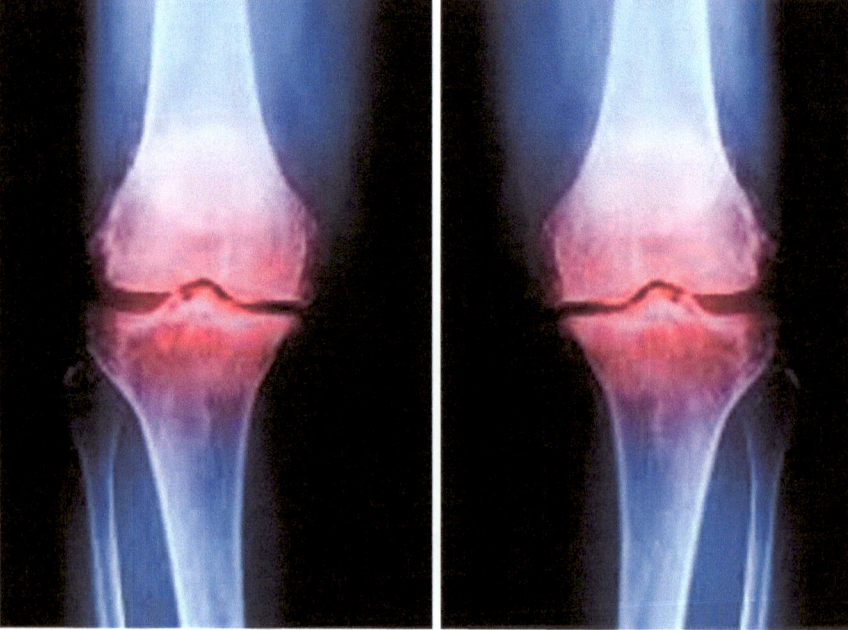

Fig. 1.2 An X-ray showing osteoarthritis

The results of radiographs do not always relate to symptoms. Some patients may have extensive joint damage with minimal symptoms, whereas other patients will have bothersome symptoms with only early changes on X-rays. It is important for the patient's symptoms to be treated as opposed to the results of the X-rays.

1.8.1.1 Computed Tomography (CT) Bone Scan Imaging
CT scanning will allow for further evaluation of the osseous structures, and soft-tissue calcification can be viewed with more detail than with radiography (X-ray imaging) (Hayashi et al. 2016).

1.8.1.2 Ultrasound Scan
Assessment of bone and cartilage tissue (e.g. meniscus) can be completed by ultrasound examination. Quantitative assessment of the thickness of cartilage and early detection of osteophyte formation can be assessed. The presence of fluid in the joint can also be evaluated (Grassi et al. 2016).

1.8.1.3 Magnetic Resonance Imaging (MRI)
MRI can detect cartilage degradation, synovitis and meniscal tears and aid in the classification of mild, moderate or severe osteoarthritis (Arden and Nevitt 2016). This investigation may be considered a 'gold standard' in the imaging of OA. This investigation allows for optimised visualisation of the different types of tissue (Hunter and Roemer 2016).

1.8.1.4 Laboratory Tests
There are no specific blood investigations which are diagnostic of OA. Synovial joint fluid aspirated from the joint and processed for analysis is usually 'clear' in colour or 'slightly yellow' in OA (Deveza et al. 2016). Fluid analysis can be used to differentiate OA from an inflammatory condition such as rheumatoid arthritis or from joint infection.

1.9 Treatments and Their Efficacy

Conservative management should be considered prior to surgical intervention.

1.9.1 Conservative Management

Three core treatments should be offered when the individual initially presents with osteoarthritis (National Institute of Clinical Excellence (NICE) 2014; Dziedzic et al. 2014). These include the following:

- Education and information, to include advice relating to pain management (Conaghan et al. 2015; Healey et al. 2016; Jordan et al. 2017; MacDonald et al. 2014)
- Exercise therapy, to improve strength, aerobic fitness and range of movement (Artese and Grubbs 2017; Arthritis Research UK 2018; Brosseau et al. 2003; Fransen et al. 2003)

Low levels of physical exercise can contribute to muscle wasting and increased body mass index (BMI) (Artese and Grubbs 2017). Stretching exercises in patients with lower limb OA have been found to have a larger effect on pain levels than paracetamol (Jordan et al. 2017).

- Weight management and information relating to diet (Basedow and Esterman 2015; Green et al. 2014; Hagen et al. 2016). All patients who are overweight should be offered advice and support to lose weight.
- Other conservative non-pharmacological interventions include the use of assistive devices and orthoses (e.g. walking aids, education about appropriate footwear and shoe insoles) (Messier et al. 2004; Stitik et al. 2005). Thermotherapy and transcutaneous nerve stimulation can also be helpful to reduce pain.

Patient expectations of conservative management should be discussed with ongoing support and review of progress (for more information on self–management, please see Chapter 12, and for more guidance on managing pain and optimising function, please refer to Chapters 7 and 10).

- Pharmacological options

Paracetamol is the drug of choice in the treatment of OA. Patient will require advice on the need to take pain relief regularly if pain is a constant feature. Topical non-steroidal anti-inflammatory drugs (NSAIDs) may be preferred over paracetamol in hand and knee OA as they may be more effective and have minimal systemic side effects. Another topical treatment that can be effective for hand and knee OA is capsaicin (National Institute of Clinical Excellence (NICE) 2014).

If paracetamol and topical NSAIDs are not effective, then the use of opioid analgesia (usually co-codamol) and oral NSAIDs can be considered. In older people, the existence of co-morbidities, especially those that impact on the cardiovascular, gastrointestinal and renal systems, often precludes the use of non-steroidal anti-inflammatory drugs (NSAIDs). If NSAIDs are used, they should be given for a limited period of time at the lowest effective dose and prescribed with a proton pump inhibitor (National Institute of Clinical Excellence (NICE) 2014).

Intra-articular corticosteroid injections can provide effective analgesic relief for a short period of time. Although it is not recommended to have these injections regularly due to the risks associated with long-term use, injections can be helpful to break the cycle of pain before the patient engages in an exercise programme.

The drugs names cited in this chapter reflect those medications used in the United Kingdom. Please refer to the drug information portal for alternative names used in the United States (https://druginfo.nim.nih.gov/drugportal/).

1.9.2 Surgical Options of Management

Surgical intervention can be considered when other interventions have failed to alleviate symptoms which are impacting on the individual's quality of life. The aim of surgical intervention is to reduce joint load on the damaged aspect of the joint (Hosie and Dickson 2000). Surgical options may be categorised into those that preserve the joint and those that replace the joint.

Preservation of the joint through resurfacing (hip joint) (National Joint Registry (NJR) 2017) and osteotomy (hip or knee) (Montalti and Affatato 2017) can be considered as opposed to total joint replacement surgery.

1.9.2.1 Hip Resurfacing

In hip resurfacing (Fig. 1.3), the weight-bearing surfaces of the hip joint are replaced with a new acetabular component within the pelvis and a metal bearing 'cap' to cover the head of the femur bone of the thigh. This procedure allows the head of the femur to be preserved (Blunn 2011). The surgeon assessment will determine individual suitability for this surgical procedure (Singh and Field 2011). This procedure is considered suitable for the younger person who is active and wishes to return to sport. There is less risk of dislocation compared to a total hip replacement procedure.

1.9.2.2 Osteotomy

Osteotomy is performed to correct joint deformity and alter the alignment of the knee or hip. This allows off-loading of body weight from the affected compartment of the joint which has been damaged from OA.

This procedure may be considered for a young middle-aged individual who is active, has healthy bone and has instability of the joint and deformity (Lim and Bartlett 2011).

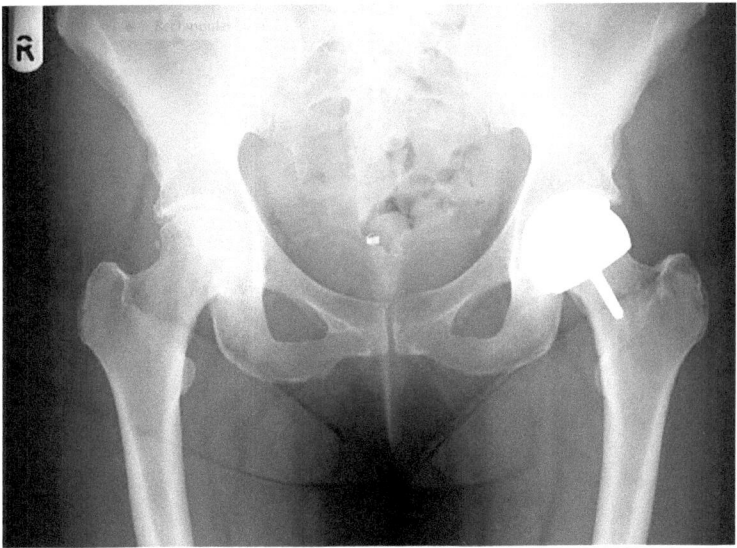

Fig. 1.3 Hip resurfacing. (With permission from Mr Philip Roberts, orthopaedic surgeon University Hospital of North Midlands. UK)

1.9.2.3 Total Joint Replacement

Total joint replacement involves a replacement of the articular surfaces of the joint (Fig. 1.4). Varying amounts of bone are removed to enable the prosthetic replacement to be fixed precisely in place (National Institute of Clinical Excellence (NICE) 2014). Hip and knee joint replacement surgery is one of the most successful interventions for treatment of pain caused by severe osteoarthritis (Hulse 2017; Srinivas and Puttaswamy 2017). This can be life changing for the individual, providing pain relief and improved mobility and overall function of the affected joint. Generally, this procedure is offered to individuals over the age of 60 years, with excellent outcomes of pain relief for 90% of patients over 10 years (Xiu and Datta 2019).

1.10   Research in Osteoarthritis

Clinical trials are ongoing, consisting of pharmacological, non-pharmacological and surgical interventions with the focus of exploring approaches to the management of symptoms and improvement in quality of life for individuals with osteoarthritis (National Institute of Health Research (NIHR) 2019). Research relating to the delivery of information to patients via telephone consultation as opposed to a face-to-face consultation has been very well received by patients (Lawford et al. 2019). In particular, the European Congress of Rheumatology (EULAR) has identified a number of OA research priorities (Felton 2014). These include the

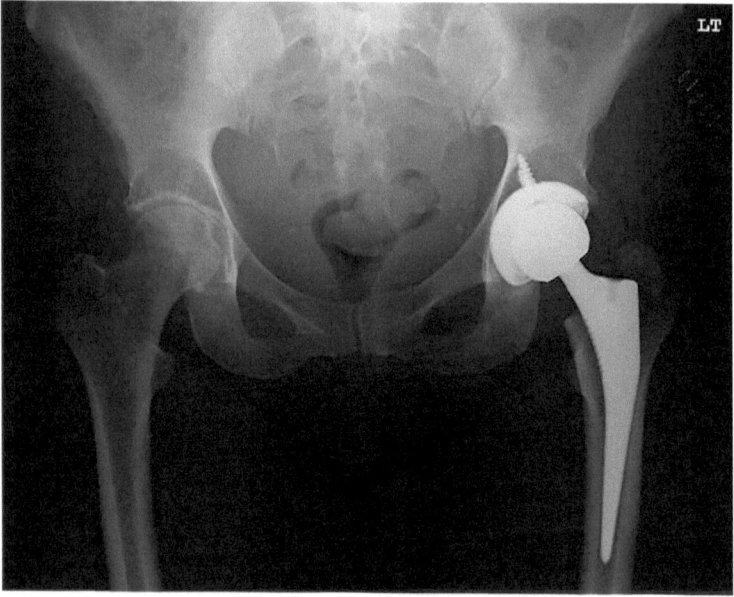

Fig. 1.4 Total hip replacement. (With permission from Mr Philip Roberts, orthopaedic surgeon University Hospital of North Midlands. UK)

mechanisms of pain in OA, treatment strategies, predictors of disease progression and a greater understanding of the effects of co-morbidities on OA pathology.

Summary of Main Points for Learning
- Osteoarthritis is a complex degenerative disease with multiple symptoms.
- Assessment and diagnosis are multifactorial.
- Self-reported tools may be used to assist the assessment process and monitor progress of the disease.
- There are three core interventions to aid the management of osteoarthritis.
- Investigations may assist in the diagnosis.
- Treatment strategies can be non-pharmacological, pharmacological and surgical.

1.11 Self-Assessment

The following are ideas of how you might relate and apply to practise what you have learnt from this chapter.

1. Discuss with a colleague how you would explain what OA is to a patient.
2. Consider how the diagnosis of OA is made and the role of investigations in supporting the diagnosis.
3. Consider how the assessment schedule could be applied to your clinical practice.
4. Discuss the conservative and surgical management of OA.

References

Allen KD, Golightly YM. Epidemiology of osteoarthritis: state of the evidence. Curr Opin Rheumatol. 2015;27(3):276–83.

Arden, Nevitt. Chapter 8: Epidemiology. In: Doherty M, Bijlsma J, Arden N, Hunter DJ, Dalbeth N, editors. Osteoarthritis and crystal arthropathy (Oxford text books in rheumatology). 3rd ed. Oxford: Oxford University Press; 2016. p. 81–90.

Artese AL, Grubbs BF. Exercise in the prevention and treatment of osteoarthritis. In: Anand A, editor. Frontiers in arthritis, vol. 1. Sharjah: Bentham Books; 2017. p. 10–22.

Arthritis Research UK. Defying arthritis together. 2018. www.arthritisresearchuk.org. Accessed 21 Apr 2019.

Basedow M, Esterman A. Assessing appropriateness of osteoarthritis care using quality indicators: a systematic review. J Eval Clin Pract. 2015;21:782–9.

Blunn. Chapter 7.6: Bearing surfaces. In: Bullstrode C, Wilson MacDonald J, Eastwood D, McMaster J, Fairbank J, Singh P, Bawa S, Gikas P, Bunker T, Giddins G, Blyth M, Stanley D, Cooke P, Carrington R, Calder P, Wordsworth P, Briggs T, editors. Trauma and orthopaedics. Oxford: Oxford University Press; 2011.

Bortoluzzi A, Furini F, Scirè CA. Osteoarthritis and its management: epidemiology, nutritional aspects, and environmental factors. Autoimmun Rev. 2018;17:1097–104.

Brosseau L, MacLeay L, Robinson V, Wells G, Tugwel P. Intensity of exercise for the treatment of osteoarthritis. Cochrane Database Syst Rev. 2003;(2):CD004259.

Canadian Hemophilia Society. Joint damage. n.d.. Retrieved from https://www.hemophilia.ca/joint-damage/.

Conaghan P, Porcheret M, Kingsbury S, Gammon A, Soni A, Hurley M, Rayman M, et al. Impact and therapy of osteoarthritis: The Arthritis Care OA Nation 2012 survey. Clin Rheumatol. 2015;34:1581–8.

Cross M, Smith E, Hoy D, Nolte S, Ackerman I, Fransen M, March L. The global burden of hip and knee osteoarthritis: estimates from the Global Burden of Disease 2010 study. Ann Rheum Dis. 2014;73(7):1323–30.

Dawson J, Fitzpatrick R, Murray D, Carr A. Questionnaire on the perceptions of patients about total knee replacement. J Bone Joint Surg Br. 1998;80(1):63–9. www.orthopaedicscores.com.

Deveza L, Ding C, Jin X, Wang X, Zhu Z, Hunter D. Chapter 19: Laboratory tests. In: Doherty, et al., editors. Osteoarthritis and crystal arthropathy. 3rd ed. Oxford: Oxford University Press; 2016. p. 191–200.

Dziedzic K, Healey E, Porcheret M, Ong B, Main C, Jordan K, Lewis M, et al. Implementing the NICE osteoarthritis guidelines: a mixed methods study and cluster randomised trial of a model osteoarthritis consultation in primary care—the management of osteoarthritis in consultations (MOSAICS) study protocol. Implement Sci. 2014;9:95.

Felton DT. Priorities for osteoarthritis research: much to be done. Nat Rev Rheumatol. 2014;10:447–8.

Fransen M, McConell S, Bell M. Exercise for osteoarthritis of the hip or knee. Cochrane Database Syst Rev. 2003;(3):CD004286.

Grassi W, Okano T, Filippucci. Chapter 17: Ultrasound in osteoarthritis and crystal related arthropathies. In: Doherty, et al., editors. Osteoarthritis and crystal arthropathy. 3rd ed. Oxford: Oxford University Press; 2016. p. 169–76.

Green J, Hirst-Jones K, Davidson R, Jupp O, et al. The potential for dietary factors to prevent or treat osteoarthritis. Proc Nutr Soc. 2014;73(2):278–88.

Greene MA, Loeser RF. Aging-related inflammation in osteoarthritis. Osteoarthr Cartil. 2015;23:1966–71.

Hagen K, Smedslund G, Osteras N, Jamtvedi G. Quality of community-based osteoarthritis care: a systematic review and meta-analysis. Arthritis Care Res (Hoboken). 2016;68(10):1443–52.

Hayashi D, Guermazi A, Roemer F. Chapter 16: Investigations for osteoarthritis: radiography and computed tomography imaging of osteoarthritis. In: Doherty, et al., editors. Osteoarthritis and crystal arthropathy. 3rd ed. Oxford: Oxford University Press; 2016. p. 157–68.

Healey E, Main C, Ryan S, McHugh G, Porcheret M, Finney A, Morden A, Dziedzic K. A nurse led clinic for patients consulting with osteoarthritis in general practice: development and impact of training in a cluster randomised controlled trial. BMC Fam Pract. 2016;17:173.

Hosie G, Dickson J. Managing osteoarthritis in primary care. Oxford: Blackwell Science; 2000.

Hulse N. Total knee replacement in arthritis – current concepts. In: Frontiers in arthritis, vol. 1. Sharjah: Bentham Books; 2017. p. 105–27.

Hunter D, Roemer F. Chapter 18: Imaging: magnetic resonance imaging. In: Doherty, et al., editors. Osteoarthritis and crystal arthropathy. 3rd ed. Oxford: Oxford University Press; 2016. p. 177.

Ickinger C, Tikly M. Current approach to diagnosis and management of osteoarthritis. S Afr Fam Pract. 2014;56(2):102–8.

Jordan K, Edwards J, Porcheret M, Healey E, Jinks C, Bedson J, Clarkson K, Hay E, Dziedzic K. Effect of a model consultation informed by guidelines on recorded quality of care of osteoarthritis (MOSAICS): a cluster randomised controlled trial in primary care. Osteoarthr Cartil. 2017;25(10):1588–97.

Laires PA, Canhão H, Rodrigues AM, Eusébio M, Gouveia M, Branco JC. The impact of osteoarthritis on early exit from work: results from a population-based study. BMC Public Health. 2018;18:472.

Lawford B, Delany C, Bennell K, Hinman R. "I Was Really Pleasantly Surprised", First-hand experience and shifts in physical therapist perceptions of telephone – delivered exercise therapy for knee osteoarthritis – a qualitative study. Arthritis Care Res. 2019;71(4):545–57.

Lim MH, Bartlett J. Chapter 8.4: Osteotomies around the knee. In: Bullstrode C, Wilson MacDonald J, Eastwood D, McMaster J, Fairbank J, Singh P, Bawa S, Gikas P, Bunker T, Giddins G, Blyth M, Stanley D, Cooke P, Carrington R, Calder P, Wordsworth P, Briggs T, editors. Trauma and orthopaedics. Oxford: Oxford University Press; 2011.

Lin E. Depression and osteoarthritis. Am J Med. 2008;121:S16–9.

MacDonald K, Sanmartin C, Langlois K, Marshall D. Symptom onset, diagnosis and management of osteoarthritis. Health Rep. 2014;25(9):10–7.

Messier SP, Loeser RF, Miller GD, Morgan TM, Rejeski WJ, Sevick MA, Ettinger WH, Pahor M, Williamson JD. Exercise and dietary weight loss in overweight and obese older adults with knee osteoarthritis: the arthritis, diet and activity promotion trial. Arthritis Rheum. 2004;50(5):1501–10.

Montalti M, Affatato S. Opening wedge osteotomies of the proximal tibia and distal femur. In: Anand A, editor. Frontiers in arthritis, vol. 1. Sharjah: Bentham Books; 2017. p. 91–104.

National Institute of Clinical Excellence (NICE). OA: Care and Management (CG 177). 2014. www.nice.org.uk/guidance/cg177.

National Institute of Health Research (NIHR). Discover the latest research. 2019. www.discover.dc.nihr.ac.uk. Accessed 04 Apr 2019.

National Joint Registry (NJR). Working for patients, driving forward quality. NJR Reports. 2017. www.njrcentre.org.uk.

O'Neill TW, McCabe PS, McBeth J. Update on the epidemiology, risk factors, and outcomes of osteoarthritis. Best Pract Res Clin Rheumatol. 2018;32:312–26.

Palazzo C, Nguyen C, Lefevre-Colau M-M, Rannou F, Poiraudeau S. Risk factors and burden of osteoarthritis. Ann Phys Rehabil Med. 2016;59:134–8.

Paterson KL, Kasza J, Hunter DJ, Hinman RS, Menz HB, Peat G, Bennell KL. The relationship between foot and ankle symptoms and risk of developing knee osteoarthritis: data from the osteoarthritis initiative. Osteoarthr Cartil. 2017;25:639–46.

Rosemann T, Laux G, Szecsenyi J, Wensing M, Grol R. Pain and osteoarthritis in primary care: factors associated with pain perception in a sample of 1,021 patients. Pain Med. 2008;9(7):903–10.

Singh, Field. Chapter 7.5: Implant choice for primary total hip replacement. In: Bullstrode C, Wilson MacDonald J, Eastwood D, McMaster J, Fairbank J, Singh P, Bawa S, Gikas P, Bunker T, Giddins G, Blyth M, Stanley D, Cooke P, Carrington R, Calder P, Wordsworth P, Briggs T, editors. Trauma and orthopaedics. Oxford: Oxford University Press; 2011.

Srinivas JV, Puttaswamy M. Total hip arthroplasty evolution and current concepts. In: Frontiers in arthritis, vol. 1. Sharjah: Bentham Books; 2017. p. 140–68.

Stitik TP, Yonclas P, Foye PM, Schoener L. Non-pharmacologic management of knee and hip osteoarthritis. J Musculoskelet Med. 2005;22:61–70.

van der Woude JAD, Nair SC, Custers RJH, van Laar JM, Kuchuck NO, Lafeber FPJG, Welsing PMJ. Knee joint distraction compared to total knee arthroplasty for treatment of end-stage osteoarthritis: simulating long-term outcomes and cost effectiveness. PLoS One. 2016;11(5):e0155524.

Xiu P, Datta S. Osteoarthritis. Rheumatology and orthopaedics. 4th ed. Amsterdam: Elsevier; 2019.

Zambon S, Siviero P, Denkinger M, Limongi F, Castell MV, van der Pas S, et al. Role of osteoarthritis, comorbidity, and pain in determining functional limitations in older populations: European Project on Osteoarthritis. Arthritis Care Res. 2016;68(6):801–10.

Further Reading

Adebajo A, Dunkley L. Chapter 9: Osteoarthritis. In: ABC of rheumatology. BMJ books. 5th ed. Hoboken, NJ: Wiley-Blackwell; 2018.

Oliver S. Chapter 2: Osteoarthritis. Oxford handbook of musculoskeletal nursing. Oxford University Press, Oxford. 2009.

Pearson S. Proactive treatment for osteoarthritis. Am Nurse Today. 2018;10:8.

Jette Primdahl and Bente Appel Esbensen

2.1   Learning Outcomes

At the end of the chapter, the nurses will be able to:

- Recognize the signs and symptoms of RA
- Describe the assessment and treatment of an older person with RA
- Understand the importance of self-management and patient education
- Identify comorbidities associated with RA

2.2   Cause

The incidence of RA varies from 0.5% to 1% in Caucasian individuals. Women are twice or three times more likely to develop RA compared to men (Smolen et al. 2018). The cause of RA is unknown and appears to involve complex associations

J. Primdahl (✉)
Danish Hospital for Rheumatic Diseases, University Hospital of Southern Denmark, Sønderborg, Denmark

Department of Regional Health Research, University of Southern Denmark, Odense, Denmark
e-mail: jprimdahl@gigtforeningen.dk

B. A. Esbensen
Copenhagen Centre for Arthritis Research, Centre for Rheumatology and Spine Diseases VRR, Head and Orthopaedics Centre, Rigshospitalet, Copenhagen, Denmark

The Department of Clinical Medicine, Faculty of Health and Medical Sciences, University of Copenhagen, Copenhagen, Denmark
e-mail: bente.appel.esbensen@regionh.dk

© Springer Nature Switzerland AG 2020
S. Ryan (ed.), *Nursing Older People with Arthritis and other Rheumatological Conditions*, Perspectives in Nursing Management and Care for Older Adults, https://doi.org/10.1007/978-3-030-18012-6_2

between genetic and environmental factors. Risk factors include a family history of RA, smoking, obesity, and genetic influences, especially in patients with antibodies toward IgG, rheumatoid factor (RF). The association between smoking and RA is linked to the presence of anti-cyclic citrullinated peptide antibodies (a-CCP).

2.3   Diagnosis

RA can occur at any age and is most commonly present in individuals 50–70 years, with a mean age of diagnosis at 61 years (Combe et al. 2017).

No specific diagnostic criteria exist for RA. The 2010 ACR/EULAR (the American and European Rheumatology Associations; American College of Rheumatology and European League Against Rheumatism) classification criteria can be used to support the diagnostic process. The criteria include joint swelling, serology (positive RF and/ or positive a-CCP, the presence of raised serum inflammatory markers (i.e., C-reactive protein), and disease duration. At least one swollen joint must be present for more than 6 weeks (Smolen et al. 2018). The diagnosis of RA is usually made on clinical evidence from the patient's history and examination. RA primarily affects the small joints in the hands and feet and is usually symmetrical in presentation. Large joint involvement includes shoulders, elbows, hips, knees, and ankles.

On clinical examination, there is often the presence of

- Joint swelling (effusions)
- Joint stiffness
- Restricted joint movement (due to swelling or joint damage)
- Muscle wasting
- Joint tenderness
- Warmth coming from a joint

Figure 2.1 shows the characteristics that are often present in patients who develop RA over the age of 65 years, when the onset of the condition is referred to as elderly onset RA.

An ultrasound scan of the hands and feet can be useful to diagnosing RA as this can detect the presence of inflammation that will not be present on a plain radiograph. X-rays can show erosions (which are usually associated with more advanced progression of RA).

When RA is suspected, the patient should be referred to see a rheumatologist as soon as possible to reduce diagnostic delay. Inflammation is considered the main

- An equal distribution between the number of men and women affected.
- A higher frequency of acute onset RA.
- Large joint involvement is more common.
- Less likelihood of having a positive rheumatoid factor.

Fig. 2.1   Characteristics of elderly onset RA

driver of the clinical symptoms, joint damage, disability, and comorbidity. Thus, a fast diagnosis and initiation of efficient pharmacological therapy are of great importance (Combe et al. 2017). In addition, older people with joint pain, joint stiffness, and joint swelling are more susceptible to develop muscle atrophy and contractions if effective pharmacological treatment is not initiated.

The serum autoantibody rheumatoid factor is seen in 50–70% of patients on diagnosis (although it is less prevalent in elderly onset RA), and if present, the RA is classified as seropositive RA. The a-CCP is also used for diagnostic purposes, and it can be positive up to 10 years before a person develops RA. For seropositive patients, the condition tends to be more severe regarding symptoms, joint damage, and increased mortality in comparison to patients who are not seropositive (Smolen et al. 2018).

2.4   The Pharmacological Treatment of RA

Pharmacological treatment aims to reduce inflammation and achieve remission (Combe et al. 2017). A treat-to-target approach is pursued, where the treatment aim is to achieve sustained remission or low disease activity in every patient (Smolen et al. 2018).

- The initial treatment for RA is conventional synthetic disease-modifying antirheumatic drugs (cDMARDS) which should be started as early as possible and ideally within 3 months after onset of symptoms (Smolen et al. 2018).
- Methotrexate is the first drug of choice and may be used in combination with low-dose glucocorticoids during the initial stages of treatment as the effect of methotrexate will only be experienced after 2–4 months (Combe et al. 2017; Smolen et al. 2017).
- The dose of methotrexate can be increased to 25–30 mg per week (depending on the national guidelines of different countries) and can be administered as tablets or subcutaneous injections.
- Parenteral administration is used if oral methotrexate is ineffective or the patients experience side effects such as nausea and other gastrointestinal symptoms.
- Treatment with methotrexate may be combined with other cDMARDS, such as sulfasalazine, hydroxychloroquine, or leflunomide (Aletaha and Smolen 2018).
- Glucocorticoids can be administered as tablets or injections and provide rapid relief of symptoms. As they have serious long-term side effects, such as osteoporosis, they are only used for short periods or in low doses.
- New biologic DMARDS (bDMARDs) target different specific modules in the inflammation process such as tumor necrosis factor (TNF) and interleukin 6 (IL6). A bDMARD is added if the patient does not respond to or is unable to tolerate cDMARDs (Combe et al. 2017).
- Rheumatology nurses have an important role in observing the effectiveness and side effects to pharmacological treatment and whether there are flares between consultations.

A substantial number of people with elderly onset RA have comorbidities or health-related problems that exclude them from taking part in drug trials. Due to the pharmacokinetic effects of aging on renal function, it is good practice to start one DMARD at a time rather than commence several DMARDs at once. Also in the older person, DMARDs can be started at a lower dose to ensure that there are no adverse effects prior to increasing the dosage to achieve an optimal response. Often older people are taking other drugs for different conditions, and the accumulative effects of all medication must be taken into account when advocating new medication to treat RA (see Chapter 9 for more information on drug therapy).

2.5   Signs, Symptoms, and Assessment

The first signs of RA will usually present as follows:

- Swollen, painful joints, and early morning joint stiffness.
- Fatigue, poor sleep, reduced physical function, and reduced quality of life.

The intensity and duration of the symptoms can vary (Hill 2006) throughout the day and from day to day, which reinforces the unpredictable nature of the disease. Patients require education and support to manage symptoms such as pain, fatigue, and sleep problems (see Chapters 6 and 7).

Figure 2.2 illustrates the nursing needs of the older people with RA.

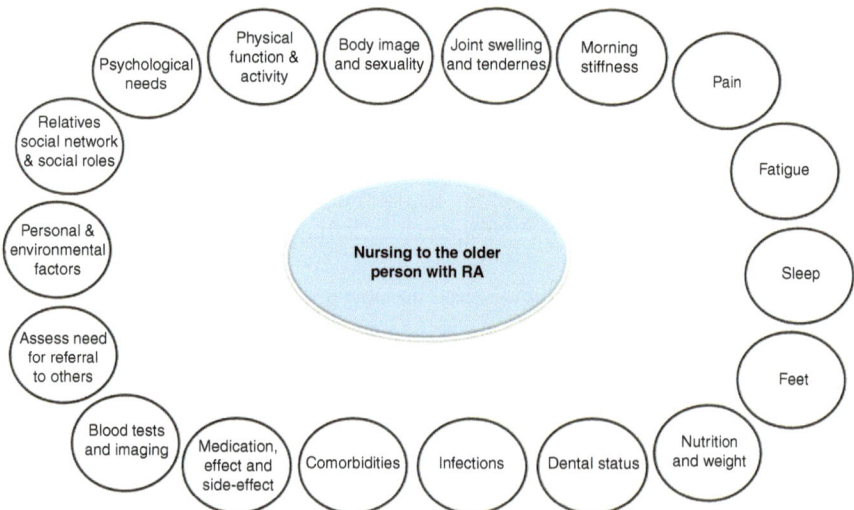

Fig. 2.2 The multidimensional nursing needs of the older people with RA

2.5.1 Pain

Pain is subjective, is difficult to measure, and can vary on a daily basis. Some patients will develop chronic widespread pain (Hill 2006). Fatigue and sleep problems are risk factors for the development of chronic widespread pain.

The management of pain involves a combination of pain-relieving medications and behavioral approaches including pacing, cognitive–behavioral therapy, and physical activity (Hill 2006). Cold therapy (including the use of ice packs) can relieve pain from swollen joints, and heat (hot shower) can help with muscle stiffness (see Chapter 7 for information on pain management).

2.5.2 Fatigue

Fatigue is highly prevalent in people with RA and is reported by 42–80% of patients, and it has a greater impact on everyday life, than pain (Hewlett et al. 2011). Pain and depression are important factors for physical, cognitive, and emotional fatigue (Feldthusen et al. 2016). RA-related fatigue is associated with reduced quality of life and poor mental health (van Hoogmoed et al. 2010). People with RA have described fatigue as overwhelming, uncontrollable, and very different from ordinary fatigue and as "a vicious circle of an unpredictable symptom" with a physical, cognitive, emotional, and social impact (Primdahl et al. 2019). Therefore, fatigue should be viewed as a complex and multifactorial subjective experience with disease related, personal, cognitive, psychological, and contextual dimensions (Hewlett et al. 2011) (see Chapter 6 for information on managing fatigue).

2.5.3 Sleep

Sixty to eighty percent of people with RA report poor sleep, in contrast to 10–30% of the general population (Loppenthin et al. 2015). Many of the symptoms older people with RA experience may be related to poor sleep quality. Sleep may be impaired due to pain, fatigue, depression, disease activity, and treatment with corticosteroids (Luyster et al. 2011; Ulus et al. 2011). In addition, poor sleep is associated with decreased quality of life, reduced self-confidence, increased fatigue, obesity, and the risk of comorbidities (Loppenthin et al. 2015; Guo et al. 2013).

Treatment of sleep problems is often based on pharmacological drugs which can lead to side effects such as tolerance, addiction, and daytime drowsiness (Jennum 2015). For older people, the use of medications may involve an increased risk of falls, fatigue, and cognitive impairment. Due to a decline in homeostatic counter regulating mechanisms that comes with aging, medications such as tricyclic antidepressants can induce hypotension and precipitate falls.

The Pittsburgh Sleep Quality Index (PSQI) (Buysse et al. 1989) is widely used to identify and assess sleep disturbances in clinical care and research. The PSQI is validated for use in patients with RA and measures sleep quality and disturbances over the prior month and differentiates between "good" and "poor" sleepers.

It is essential that the nurse explores and discusses any issues with sleep and possible associations to fatigue, pain, and physical activity with the patient.

Advice the nurse can provide on improving sleep include establishing a sleep routine (settling at the same time each night), ensuring that the bedroom is well ventilated, undertaking regular exercise, and avoiding caffeine-based drinks and alcohol in the evening.

2.6 Management

The management of RA has changed during the past years due to the development of new effective therapies. Nurses have an important role in disease management (Combe et al. 2017; Bech et al. 2019). Pharmacological treatment should be initiated as soon as possible, as early effective treatment leads to better outcomes for the patient in terms of remission and less joint damage (Combe et al. 2017). The nurse has a major role in educating and supporting the patient to manage the symptoms of RA (Barlow et al. 1999).

Apart from self-management (see Chapter 12) and patient education, nonpharmacological interventions encompassing physical therapy, occupational therapy, and health promotion can be addressed as part of a rehabilitation process. Rehabilitation is defined by the World Health Organization as "a set of measures that assist individuals, who experience or are likely to experience disability, to achieve and maintain optimum functioning in interaction with their environments" (World Health Organization 2014) (p. 3). Rehabilitation is based on a biopsychosocial approach where the focus is on the patients' physical, psychological and social function, and functional limitations, rather than the diagnosis. The same diagnosis can lead to very different limitations and challenges for the individual person. In the same way, physiological aging differs, and the patient's chronological age does not always relate to functional level.

Personal factors (i.e., the persons' educational background, motivation, experiences, life goals, and values) and environmental factors (i.e., housing, family, and whether there are stairs to climb) affect how individuals function on a daily basis and whether or how they are able to participate in family and social activities. These factors must be taken into consideration when planning care that will have meaning and relevance for the older patient (Taylor and Geyh 2012).

2.6.1 Patient Education

People with RA do not always take their medicine as prescribed, and it is important to discuss their beliefs about the illness and the medication as education can increase adherence (de Thurah et al. 2010; Ritschl et al. 2018).

- Patients should be offered individually tailored education from the multidisciplinary team about RA, what signs and symptoms to expect, and how to manage them. When new medications are prescribed and whenever the individual patient experience a need for education, the patient should be offered education (Zangi et al. 2015).
- Patient education can be offered by the nurse face-to-face, in groups, on the telephone or online (Zangi et al. 2015).
- Educational aspects include pharmacological treatment, management of pain, sleep and fatigue, living well with a chronic condition, smoking cessation, dental care, weight control, vaccination, and comorbidities (Combe et al. 2017; Zangi et al. 2015).

Nurses should be offered and undertake education to build their own competence regarding providing patient education (Zangi et al. 2015). It is important that the members in the team know the competences each different health professional has and that there is communication and dialogue between the team members to ensure coherent care.

2.6.2 Physical Activity, Physical Therapy, and Occupational Therapy

In general, people with RA are less physically active than people without RA. People with RA reduce their physical activity (PA) level by two thirds after being diagnosed, and the activities they maintain tend to be at a lower level compared to before diagnosis (Sokka et al. 2008). This may be due to disease-related factors such as pain, fatigue, sleep, and functional limitations. At the same time, PA has a positive effect on pain, fatigue, sleep, and general well-being (Thomsen et al. 2017). All nurses should be able to provide general advice regarding PA (see Chapter 10). Furthermore, the nurse can explore potential barriers for PA. Some patients are afraid that PA may lead to an aggravation of the condition (Rausch Osthoff et al. 2018). It is important to support the patient based on their individual goals and to start with light PA and increase the level gradually, especially if the patient has not been physically active for some time (Rausch Osthoff et al. 2018).

Older patients, with comorbidities, may require referring to a physiotherapist or an occupational therapist for assessment and specific guidance and training in relation to individual problems and to incorporate other health-related needs, for example, cardiac problems into their care management. Apart from specific problems with movement and physical activity, the physiotherapist can offer advice on increased aerobic capacity, strength, and balance. Occupational therapists can assess and support the older patient to remain independent when carrying out daily activities and encourage social participation. Other health professionals involved in the patient's care may include a dietician, a psychologist, podiatrist, or a social worker.

2.6.3 Psychosocial Support

Patients respond differently to being diagnosed with RA. For some, it is a relief finally to receive a diagnosis and an explanation for various symptoms (Kostova et al. 2014). Other individuals experience grief due to activities that can no longer be managed (Ryan 2006) and experience a changed perception of their own identity and body image. RA can also impact on body image, sexuality, and roles within the family (Kristiansen et al. 2012; Helland et al. 2011).

According to European recommendations, nurses should address psychosocial issues such as anxiety and depression (van Eijk-Hustings et al. 2012). The nurse can address how the condition has impacted on the patients' well-being and assess the varying need for psychological and emotional support (Ryan 2006) (see Chapter 8 for more information on psychological and social impact of arthritis).

2.6.4 Outpatient Follow-Up

In clinical practice, when the patient attends an outpatient follow-up, the rheumatologist or the nurse will examine the number of tender and swollen joints on the hands, wrists, elbows, shoulders, and knees. Often, the joints in the feet are examined as well. Problems with the feet will affect the patient's mobility (see Chapter 11). Together with the CRP or erythrocyte sedimentation rate (ESR) and the patient's global assessment of disease impact on a VAS scale, a composite score, the Disease Activity Score, is calculated (DAS28-CRP or DAS28-ESR) (Fransen and van Riel 2005). The global impact of RA is assessed on a VAS scale by both the clinician and the patient (Combe et al. 2017). The patient will complete a questionnaire on physical function (The Health Assessment Questionnaire (HAQ) (Bruce and Fries 2005)) to monitor changes over time. Approximately every 2 years, X-rays of hands and feet are required to monitor for the progression of erosions in the joints. DXA scans are used to monitor bone density.

Traditionally, patients with RA were offered an outpatient follow-up by a physician, but nurse-led follow-up is effective in achieving disease control and patient satisfaction (de Thurah et al. 2017; Primdahl et al. 2012). Due to the unpredictable nature of the disease, planned consultations may be at a time, where the patient is not experiencing any problems. Thus, patient-initiated follow-up, where the patients do not have planned consultations apart from a yearly visit, have been developed. This type of outpatient follow-up showed similar results to physician-led follow-up regarding disease control (Hewlett et al. 2005; Primdahl et al. 2014). During the past years, a simple form of tight monitoring by patient reported outcomes and tele-health was tested too (de Thurah et al. 2018). Physicians or nurses called the patient for a telephone consultation every 3–4 months after they had completed different questionnaires online. Telephone consultations, which might be more appropriate for the older person, who finds it physically difficult to attend for an outpatient appointment, have shown similar positive results regarding disease control to traditional outpatient follow-up (de Thurah et al. 2018).

2.7   Comorbidities Associated with the Condition

Older people with RA have an increased prevalence of comorbidities, such as cardiovascular disease, infections, certain types of cancer, osteoporosis, peptic ulcer, and depression (Baillet et al. 2016). Inflammation is associated with secondary amyloidosis, lymphoma and cardiovascular disease, and thus an overall increased mortality (Smolen et al. 2016). In addition, patients with RA can develop various extra-articular manifestations, including vasculitis, interstitial lung disease, and nodules (Smolen et al. 2016).

Patients with comorbidities have a higher risk of functional decline, and thus, it is important to screen for and support older patients to prevent and manage their comorbidities (Dougados 2016; Dougados et al. 2014). As part of the rheumatology team, nurses have an important role to help detect and ensure management of comorbidities (Baillet et al. 2016).

Many comorbidities can impact functional ability in the older person. The process of aging reduces muscle mass, which can make walking difficult. It is important to support the older person to engage in light intensity and short-duration physical activities as any form of activity will reduce the rate of functional decline in older people.

2.7.1   Cardiovascular Disease

People with RA have an increased risk of cardiovascular (CV) disease similar to the CV risk for people with diabetes mellitus (Agca et al. 2017). This is due to the presence of inflammation and an increased incidence of certain risk factors for CV disease, including obesity, low high-density lipoprotein cholesterol, high low-density lipoprotein cholesterol, and low physical activity (Primdahl et al. 2013). Screening for CV risk is recommended at least every 5 years and more often in people at high risk (Agca et al. 2017).

Rheumatology nurses have an important role in discussing weight management, diet, physical activity, smoking, and alcohol habits in the older person with RA (Primdahl et al. 2016).

2.7.2   Vaccinations

Vaccination status should be assessed at diagnosis, and recommendations regarding further vaccinations should be discussed with each patient (van Assen et al. 2011; Westra et al. 2015). Patients treated with anti-TNF and corticosteroids have the highest risk for infections, and RA also poses a risk for herpes zoster with older people having an increased risk of herpes zoster independent of having RA (Westra et al. 2015). Older patients also have an increased risk of hospital admission for pneumonia or influenza. The influenza vaccination is recommended for all patients with RA and especially older people, as it can reduce the incidence of pneumonitis, acute bronchitis, and viral infections (Westra et al. 2015). Treatment with methotrexate, anti-TNF, and rituximab can reduce the efficacy of the vaccine (Westra et al. 2015).

2.7.3 Osteoporosis

Rheumatology nurses should be aware of the patients' increased risk of osteoporosis and the potential risk of falls in older people with RA. Low body mass index, physical inactivity, treatment with glucocorticoids, high alcohol intake, and a family history of osteoporosis increase the risk of osteoporosis and osteoporotic fractures (Baillet et al. 2016). Older patients should have their serum vitamin D levels checked, as vitamin D is important for bone density and muscle strength. According to European guidance, patients at an increased risk of osteoporosis should be treated with calcium and D-vitamin daily (Kanis et al. 2019). Depending on bone density, further treatment with bisphosphonates may be relevant, and the patient will need specific instructions regarding how to take this medication (see Chapter 5).

Older patients have an increased risk for the development of additional chronic diseases, such as diabetes, osteoarthritis, chronic pulmonary lung disease, and cancer. Thus, rheumatology nurses should be aware of the general signs and symptoms of these comorbidities in older people with RA.

Summary of Main Points for Learning

- RA is a chronic inflammatory disease primarily affecting the small joints of the hands and feet.
- Common symptoms are reduced mobility, pain, fatigue, stiffness of the joints, sleep problems, and depression.
- Effective pharmacological treatment is initiated as soon as possible to prevent joint damage and cardiovascular disease among others.
- It is important to monitor disease activity as well as disease impact and be aware of the importance of personal and environmental factors.
- Rheumatology nurses have an important role in disease management, which includes enhancement of the patient's self-management ability through patient education and support, and referral to other health professionals when needed.
- Management of older people with RA is a permanent challenge due to wide heterogeneity in terms of clinical presentation, treatment response, comorbidities, and physiological decline.
- Rheumatology nurses need to perform a multidimensional health and functional assessment of the patient.

2.8 Self-Assessment

Assessing your own learning and performance needs regarding the management of the older person with RA. Having read the chapter and undertaken further study, the following are some ideas to as how to relate what you have learnt to your practice.

1. Describe the clinical signs you would expect to see in a person with newly diagnosed RA.
2. Discuss with a colleague what investigations can be used to aid the diagnosis of RA.
3. Consider how you can help to support self-management in an older person with RA.
4. Discuss with your colleagues how you would explain the purpose of drug therapy to an older person.
5. Identify common comorbidities in older people with RA.

References

Agca R, Heslinga SC, Rollefstad S, Heslinga M, McInnes IB, Peters MJ, et al. EULAR recommendations for cardiovascular disease risk management in patients with rheumatoid arthritis and other forms of inflammatory joint disorders: 2015/2016 update. Ann Rheum Dis. 2017;76(1):17–28.

Aletaha D, Smolen JS. Diagnosis and management of rheumatoid arthritis: a review. JAMA. 2018;320(13):1360–72.

van Assen S, Agmon-Levin N, Elkayam O, Cervera R, Doran MF, Dougados M, et al. EULAR recommendations for vaccination in adult patients with autoimmune inflammatory rheumatic diseases. Ann Rheum Dis. 2011;70(3):414–22.

Baillet A, Gossec L, Carmona L, Wit M, van Eijk-Hustings Y, Bertheussen H, et al. Points to consider for reporting, screening for and preventing selected comorbidities in chronic inflammatory rheumatic diseases in daily practice: a EULAR initiative. Ann Rheum Dis. 2016;75(6):965–73.

Barlow JH, Cullen LA, Rowe IF. Comparison of knowledge and psychological well-being between patients with a short disease duration (< or = 1 year) and patients with more established rheumatoid arthritis (> or = 10 years duration). Patient Educ Couns. 1999;38(3):195–203.

Bruce B, Fries JF. The Health Assessment Questionnaire (HAQ). Clin Exp Rheumatol. 2005;23(5 Suppl 39):S14–8.

Buysse DJ, Reynolds CF, Monk TH, Berman SR, Kupfer DJ. The Pittsburgh Sleep Quality Index: a new instrument for psychiatric practice and research. Psychiatry Res. 1989;28(2):193–213.

Combe B, Landewe R, Daien CI, Hua C, Aletaha D, Alvaro-Gracia JM, et al. 2016 update of the EULAR recommendations for the management of early arthritis. Ann Rheum Dis. 2017;76(6):948–59.

Dougados M. Comorbidities in rheumatoid arthritis. Curr Opin Rheumatol. 2016;28(3):282–8.

Dougados M, Soubrier M, Antunez A, Balint P, Balsa A, Buch MH, et al. Prevalence of comorbidities in rheumatoid arthritis and evaluation of their monitoring: results of an international, cross-sectional study (COMORA). Ann Rheum Dis. 2014;73(1):62–8.

Bech B, Primdahl J, van Tubergen A, et al. 2018 update of the EULAR recommendations for the role of the nurse in the management of chronic inflammatory arthritis. Ann Rheum Dis. 2019; https://doi.org/10.1136/annrheumdis-2019-215458. pii: annrheumdis-2019-215458. [Epub ahead of print] van Eijk-Hustings Y, van Tubergen A, Bostrom C, Braychenko E, Buss B, Felix J, et al. EULAR recommendations for the role of the nurse in the management of chronic inflammatory arthritis. Ann Rheum Dis. 2012;71(1):13–9.

Feldthusen C, Grimby-Ekman A, Forsblad-d'Elia H, Jacobsson L, Mannerkorpi K. Explanatory factors and predictors of fatigue in persons with rheumatoid arthritis: a longitudinal study. J Rehabil Med. 2016;48(5):469–76.

Fransen J, van Riel PL. The Disease Activity Score and the EULAR response criteria. Clin Exp Rheumatol. 2005;23(5 Suppl 39):S93–9.

Guo X, Zheng L, Wang J, Zhang X, Zhang X, Li J, et al. Epidemiological evidence for the link between sleep duration and high blood pressure: a systematic review and meta-analysis. Sleep Med. 2013;14(4):324–32.

Helland Y, Kjeken I, Steen E, Kvien TK, Hauge MI, Dagfinrud H. Rheumatic diseases and sexuality: disease impact and self-management strategies. Arthritis Care Res. 2011;63(5):743–50.

Hewlett S, Kirwan J, Pollock J, Mitchell K, Hehir M, Blair PS, et al. Patient initiated outpatient follow up in rheumatoid arthritis: six year randomised controlled trial. BMJ. 2005;330(7484):171.

Hewlett S, Chalder T, Choy E, Cramp F, Davis B, Dures E, et al. Fatigue in rheumatoid arthritis: time for a conceptual model. Rheumatology (Oxford). 2011;50(6):1004–6.

Hill J. Pain and stiffness. In: Hill J, editor. Rheumatology nursing: a creative approach. 2nd ed. West Sussex, UK: John Wiley & Sons, Ltd; 2006.

van Hoogmoed D, Fransen J, Bleijenberg G, van Riel P. Physical and psychosocial correlates of severe fatigue in rheumatoid arthritis. Rheumatology (Oxford). 2010;49(7):1294–302.

Jennum P. Søvn og sundhed (Sleep and health). Report. 2015.

Kanis JA, Cooper C, Rizzoli R, Reginster JY. Executive summary of the European guidance for the diagnosis and management of osteoporosis in postmenopausal women. Calcif Tissue Int. 2019;104(3):235–8.

Kostova Z, Caiata-Zufferey M, Schulz PJ. The process of acceptance among rheumatoid arthritis patients in Switzerland: a qualitative study. Pain Res Manag. 2014;19(2):61–8.

Kristiansen TM, Primdahl J, Antoft R, Horslev-Petersen K. Everyday life with rheumatoid arthritis and implications for patient education and clinical practice: a focus group study. Musculoskeletal Care. 2012;10(1):29–38.

Loppenthin K, Esbensen BA, Ostergaard M, Jennum P, Tolver A, Aadahl M, et al. Physical activity and the association with fatigue and sleep in Danish patients with rheumatoid arthritis. Rheumatol Int. 2015;35(10):1655–64.

Luyster FS, Chasens ER, Wasko MC, Dunbar-Jacob J. Sleep quality and functional disability in patients with rheumatoid arthritis. J Clin Sleep Med. 2011;7(1):49–55.

Primdahl J, Wagner L, Holst R, Horslev-Petersen K. The impact on self-efficacy of different types of follow-up care and disease status in patients with rheumatoid arthritis—a randomized trial. Patient Educ Couns. 2012;88(1):121–8.

Primdahl J, Clausen J, Horslev-Petersen K. Results from systematic screening for cardiovascular risk in outpatients with rheumatoid arthritis in accordance with the EULAR recommendations. Ann Rheum Dis. 2013;72(11):1771–6.

Primdahl J, Sorensen J, Horn HC, Petersen R, Horslev-Petersen K. Shared care or nursing consultations as an alternative to rheumatologist follow-up for rheumatoid arthritis outpatients with low disease activity—patient outcomes from a 2-year, randomised controlled trial. Ann Rheum Dis. 2014;73(2):357–64.

Primdahl J, Ferreira RJ, Garcia-Diaz S, Ndosi M, Palmer D, van Eijk-Hustings Y. Nurses' role in cardiovascular risk assessment and management in people with inflammatory arthritis: a European perspective. Musculoskeletal Care. 2016;14(3):133–51.

Primdahl J, Hegelund A, Lorenzen AG, Loeppenthin K, Dures E, Appel Esbensen B. The experience of people with rheumatoid arthritis living with fatigue: a qualitative metasynthesis. BMJ Open. 2019;9(3):e024338.

Rausch Osthoff AK, Niedermann K, Braun J, Adams J, Brodin N, Dagfinrud H, et al. 2018 EULAR recommendations for physical activity in people with inflammatory arthritis and osteoarthritis. Ann Rheum Dis. 2018;77(9):1251–60.

Ritschl V, Lackner A, Bostrom C, Mosor E, Lehner M, Omara M, et al. I do not want to suppress the natural process of inflammation: new insights on factors associated with non-adherence in rheumatoid arthritis. Arthritis Res Ther. 2018;20(1):234.

Ryan S. The psychological aspects of rheumatic disease. In: Hill J, editor. Rheumatology nursing: a creative approach. 2nd ed. John Wiley & Sons, Ltd: West Sussex, UK; 2006.

Smolen JS, Aletaha D, McInnes IB. Rheumatoid arthritis. Lancet. 2016;388(10055):2023–38.

Smolen JS, Landewe R, Bijlsma J, Burmester G, Chatzidionysiou K, Dougados M, et al. EULAR recommendations for the management of rheumatoid arthritis with synthetic and biological disease-modifying antirheumatic drugs: 2016 update. Ann Rheum Dis. 2017;76(6):960–77.

Smolen JS, Aletaha D, Barton A, Burmester GR, Emery P, Firestein GS, et al. Rheumatoid arthritis. Nat Rev Dis Primers. 2018;4:18001.

Sokka T, Hakkinen A, Kautiainen H, Maillefert JF, Toloza S, Mork Hansen T, et al. Physical inactivity in patients with rheumatoid arthritis: data from twenty-one countries in a cross-sectional, international study. Arthritis Rheum. 2008;59(1):42–50.

Taylor WJ, Geyh S. A rehabilitation framework: the International Classification of Functioning, Disability and Health. In: Sareh G, Dean RJSWJT, editors. Interprofessional rehabilitation: a person-centred approach. West Sussex, UK: John Wiley & Sons, Ltd; 2012.

Thomsen T, Aadahl M, Beyer N, Hetland ML, Loppenthin K, Midtgaard J, et al. The efficacy of motivational counselling and SMS reminders on daily sitting time in patients with rheumatoid arthritis: a randomised controlled trial. Ann Rheum Dis. 2017;76(9):1603–6.

de Thurah A, Norgaard M, Harder I, Stengaard-Pedersen K. Compliance with methotrexate treatment in patients with rheumatoid arthritis: influence of patients' beliefs about the medicine. A prospective cohort study. Rheumatol Int. 2010;30(11):1441–8.

de Thurah A, Esbensen BA, Roelsgaard IK, Frandsen TF, Primdahl J. Efficacy of embedded nurse-led versus conventional physician-led follow-up in rheumatoid arthritis: a systematic review and meta-analysis. RMD Open. 2017;3(2):e000481.

de Thurah A, Stengaard-Pedersen K, Axelsen M, Fredberg U, Schougaard LMV, Hjollund NHI, et al. Tele-health follow up strategy for tight control of disease activity in rheumatoid arthritis: results of a randomized controlled trial. Arthritis Care Res. 2018;70(3):353–60.

Ulus Y, Akyol Y, Tander B, Durmus D, Bilgici A, Kuru O. Sleep quality in fibromyalgia and rheumatoid arthritis: associations with pain, fatigue, depression, and disease activity. Clin Exp Rheumatol. 2011;29(6 Suppl 69):S92–6.

Westra J, Rondaan C, van Assen S, Bijl M. Vaccination of patients with autoimmune inflammatory rheumatic diseases. Nat Rev Rheumatol. 2015;11(3):135–45.

World Health Organization. CONCEPT PAPER. WHO Guidelines on Health-Related Rehabilitation (Rehabilitation Guidelines). WHO; 2014.

Zangi HA, Ndosi M, Adams J, Andersen L, Bode C, Bostrom C, et al. EULAR recommendations for patient education for people with inflammatory arthritis. Ann Rheum Dis. 2015;74(6):954–62.

Further Reading

Kobak S, Bes C. An autumn tale: geriatric RA. Ther Adv Musculoskelet Dis. 2018;10(1):3–11. Access at https://www.ncbi.nlm.nih.gov/pmc/articles/PMC5724645/.

Lahaye C, Tatar Z, Dubost JJ, et al. Management of inflammatory rheumatic conditions in the elderly. Rheumatology. 2019;58(5):748–64. Access at https://academic.oup.com/rheumatology/article/58/5/748/5048710.

van Onna M, Ozturk B, Sharmens M, et al. Disease and management beliefs of elderly people with rheumatoid arthritis and co-morbidity: a qualitative study. Clin Rheumatol. 2018;37(9):2367–72. Access at https://academic.oup.com/rheumatology/article/48/12/1575/1786963.

Gout

3

Andrew Finney and Edward Roddy

3.1 Learning Outcomes

At the end of this chapter, nurses will be able to:

1. Provide a good explanation of gout
2. Understand how gout is diagnosed
3. Recognise the different pharmacological interventions for gout
4. Understand the patient lifestyle needs

3.2 Introduction

People commonly think of gout as a disease of the past, a 'rich man's disease' caused by a rich diet, obesity and overconsumption of alcohol—evoking stereotypical images of historical figures such as King Henry VIII (Richardson et al. 2016). This negative and incorrect perception of gout as a condition with an historical link to a life of dissipation leads to underestimating the prevalence and impact of this form of inflammatory arthritis (Punzi 2017). Gout is most often characterised by recurrent sudden acute flares of excruciating joint pain, swelling and inflammation.

A. Finney (✉)
School of Primary, Community and Social Care, Keele University, Staffordshire, UK

School of Nursing and Midwifery, Keele University, Staffordshire, UK
e-mail: a.finney@keele.ac.uk

E. Roddy
School of Primary, Community and Social Care, Keele University, Staffordshire, UK

Haywood Academic Rheumatology Centre, Haywood Hospital, Midlands Partnership NHS Foundation Trust, Staffordshire, UK

© Springer Nature Switzerland AG 2020
S. Ryan (ed.), *Nursing Older People with Arthritis and other Rheumatological Conditions*, Perspectives in Nursing Management and Care for Older Adults,
https://doi.org/10.1007/978-3-030-18012-6_3

Poorly managed gout can cause disabling joint damage and is associated with multiple comorbidities (renal impairment, metabolic syndrome, heart disease and depression) (Rees and Doherty 2014).

The prevalence of gout is on the increase worldwide and now affects 2.5% of the adult population in the United Kingdom and 4% in the United States, making it the most common form of inflammatory arthritis (Kuo et al. 2015; Abhishek et al. 2017). It is four times more common in men than in women and is more common in older ages; prevalence peaks between the ages of 80–84 where it affects up to 15% of men and 6% of women (Rees and Doherty 2014).

Generally, patients are managed in primary care general practice through lifestyle and drug therapy approaches. However, despite gout being considered to be the only curable form of arthritis (Rees and Doherty 2014) and there being inexpensive and well-tolerated drug treatments available, primary care management for gout has been shown to be sub-optimal and not concordant with current national and international recommendations (Rees and Doherty 2014). In view of this, new approaches are required to improve the management of gout and nurses can play a key part in this.

3.3 Defining Gout

Historically, gout has been viewed as an episodic acute inflammatory condition. It is now considered to be a chronic inflammatory arthritis, and it is more specifically a disease characterised as a long-term condition and an intensely painful form of inflammatory arthritis caused by the formation of needle-shaped chronic monosodium urate crystal deposition (Bursill et al. 2019). Gout results from sustained elevated serum urate (often reported as serum uric acid (sUA)) levels (hyperuricaemia) beyond a saturation point which leads to the formation and deposition of monosodium urate crystals in and around the joint. Crystal deposition causes sudden inflammatory flares, chronic erosive joint damage and subcutaneous deposits of urate crystals (tophi).

3.4 Risk Factors

Myths and misconceptions that hyperuricaemia and gout is simply caused by excessive amounts of alcohol and over-eating and obesity do not tell the whole story. However, risk factors (Box 3.1) for gout include obesity; excess consumption of beer or spirits, red meat, seafood, fructose-sweetened beverages and fruit juices; in many patients gout is due to genetic factors; comorbid medical conditions such as hypertension, chronic kidney disease and obstructive sleep apnoea; or some medications (particularly diuretics) rather than lifestyle factors (Roddy and Choi 2014).

Hyperuricaemia can arise from over-production or renal under-excretion of urate (Abhishek et al. 2017). Renal under-excretion is much more common, accounting for hyperuricaemia in over 90% of people with gout.

Box 3.1 Clinically Important Risk Factors for Gout (Roddy et al. 2013)
Male gender
  Older age
  Genetics
  Obesity
  Hypertension
  Hyperlipidaemia
  Use of diuretics
  Chronic kidney disease
  Metabolic syndrome
  Osteoarthritis
  Diet
  —Excess purine-rich foods, fructose, sugar-sweetened soft drinks and alcoholic drinks, particularly beer

3.5 Signs and Symptoms of Gout

Gout flares present as severe acute joint pain, with swelling (Fig. 3.1), erythema (reddening of the skin), difficulty moving the affected joint and extreme joint tenderness (Dalbeth et al. 2016). Flares typically come on rapidly, reaching peak pain intensity within 12–24 hours of onset. They commonly occur at night with patients reporting loss of sleep due to the pain and the inability to withstand even bedding touching the tender joint. Triggers for flares include acute medical or surgical illness, dehydration or dietary binges, although commonly no trigger is identified (Dalbeth et al. 2016).

3.6 Diagnosing Gout

Gout mainly affects men aged 40 years and over and women over the age of 65 (Roddy et al. 2013). Gout can run in families due to lifestyle and genetic factors.

Over time, monosodium urate crystals form in and around the joints and can eventually trigger an acute gout flare. Such flares usually present with an excruciatingly painful, red, hot and swollen joint(s). The skin often appears tight and shiny (Roddy et al. 2013). Patients will report the rapidity of acute flares that come on typically during the night, peaking within 12–24 hours and usually subsiding within 1–2 weeks (Abhishek et al. 2017). Gout most commonly affects the first metatarsophalangeal (MTP) joint (the big toe), but it can also affect the midfoot, ankle, knee, elbows or hands (Versus Arthritis 2019). It usually affects a single joint (monoarticular gout) at a time, but multiple joints can be affected at once (polyarticular gout). Monosodium urate crystals can also form outside of the joint and under the skin forming white hard lumps called tophi (Fig. 3.1) (Versus Arthritis 2019).

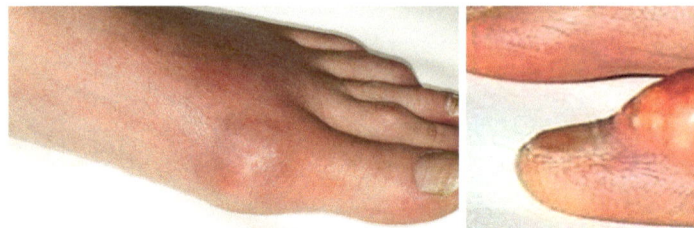

Fig. 3.1 Joint swelling and tophi

Making the diagnosis clinically is most often based on symptoms, clinical history and an examination of the affected joint. An acute flare in one joint with excruciating pain, swelling and redness that peaks within 24 hours is highly characteristics of gout, particularly when the first MTP joint is affected (Rees and Doherty 2014). When diagnostic uncertainty exists, joint aspiration and microscopy of synovial fluid can identify monosodium urate crystals, making a definitive diagnosis. Although the serum urate level is elevated in people with gout, it should be noted that serum urate on its own is not a useful diagnostic test as most people with hyperuricaemia do not have gout and serum urate can be falsely low when measured during an acute flare (Rees and Doherty 2014).

Comorbidity screening is important; a blood test can be requested for urea and electrolytes, estimated glomerular filtration rate, glucose and lipids. Addressing the problems of raised blood pressure, raised body mass index, smoking and alcohol use, along with cardiovascular risk should form part of a comprehensive patient assessment (Roddy et al. 2013). Plain X-rays have a limited role and are frequently normal in early disease (Roddy et al. 2013). Differential diagnoses include other crystal arthritides (such as calcium pyrophosphate crystal deposition (pseudo gout)), septic arthritis and reactive arthritis (Abhishek et al. 2017; Zhang et al. 2006a).

3.7 Gout and Associated Comorbidities

Gout should be viewed as more than just an inflammatory disease of the joints. Comorbidities are common place. A US National Health and Nutrition Examination Survey from 2008 showed that 74% of people with gout had hypertension, 71% had stage 2 or greater chronic kidney disease, 53% were obese, 26% had diabetes, 14% had had a myocardial infarction, and 10% had a history of stroke (Zhu et al. 2012). Sleep apnoea is also a risk factor for gout (Bucknall et al. 2018). At its worst, gout is associated with earlier mortality due to links with cardiovascular disease (Zhu et al. 2012). Gout has, however, been associated with reduced risk of neurological disorders such as Parkinson's disease, Alzheimer's and dementia (Dalbeth et al. 2016). These comorbidities can adversely affect diagnosis, make management choices difficult and contribute to long-term adverse clinical outcomes (Roddy et al. 2013).

3.8 Treatments for Gout

Although pharmacological treatments for gout are the gold standard approach, nurses need to be aware that lifestyle advice and positive lifestyle changes should form part of the patient management plan.

3.8.1 Urate Lowering Therapy (ULT)

ULT is the main component of curative gout therapy and should adopt a 'treat to target' approach for reduction of sUA. The British Society for Rheumatology guideline recommends upward titration of ULT to lower serum urate below a therapeutic target of 300 μmol/l, in order to enable dissolution of crystals to prevent flares, prevent long-term joint damage, shrink tophi and, in effect, cure gout (Rees et al. 2014; Hui et al. 2017).

3.8.1.1 Allopurinol
Allopurinol is by far the most commonly used ULT in the United Kingdom and most other countries. It is a purine analogue and a non-specific competitive inhibitor of xanthine oxidase, thereby reducing the production of uric acid (Rees et al. 2014). With the dose range of allopurinol being large (100–900 mg), this allows for it to be titrated in small increments until its effect is maximised. It is usually commenced at low dose (100 mg daily). The serum urate level should be checked 1 month after each dose change, and the daily dose increased by a further 100 mg each month until the therapeutic target serum urate level below 300 μmol/l is reached, up to the maximum dose of 900 mg daily. Allopurinol is usually well tolerated, but side-effects include nausea, gastrointestinal problems, headache and rash (Rees et al. 2014). Rarely, allopurinol can cause a life-threatening hypersensitivity syndrome which is more common in people with chronic kidney disease. For this reason, more cautious dose escalation is required in people with chronic kidney disease.

3.8.1.2 Febuxostat
Most patients can be successfully treated with allopurinol. Febuxostat has been approved by the National Institute for Health and Care Excellence (NICE) for the treatment of gout in patients who do not tolerate allopurinol. It is a non-purine, highly specific xanthine oxidase inhibitor that undergoes hepatic metabolism and, hence, does not require dose reduction in chronic kidney disease (Rees et al. 2014). It is available in two licensed doses—initially 80 mg daily which can then be increased to 120 mg daily after 1 month if the target serum urate level is not achieved. Febuxostat is a more potent urate-lowering drug than allopurinol, and both licensed doses produce larger reductions in the serum urate level than fixed-dose allopurinol 300 mg daily (Becker et al. 2005). However, febuxostat may be associated with greater cardiovascular risk than allopurinol, and hence, it is not recommended by NICE or the European Medicines Agency for use in patients with ischaemic heart disease or congestive cardiac failure.

3.8.1.3 Uricosuric Drugs

Uricosuric drugs prevent the reuptake of uric acid and, therefore, increase its excretion renally. They are used uncommonly outside specialist centres but provide a useful therapeutic option in patients who are unable to tolerate, have contraindications to or do not fully respond to allopurinol and/or febuxostat. There are three uricosuric drugs available in the United Kingdom: benzbromarone (50–200 mg daily), sulfinpyrazone (200–800 mg daily) and probenecid (250–500 mg twice daily).

3.8.1.4 Flare Prophylaxis

Initiation or increasing the dose of any urate-lowering therapy can trigger a gout flare because partial crystal dissolution occurs as a result of urate-lowering. The greater the extent of urate-lowering, the greater the risk of a flare; hence, the risk is greatest with febuxostat. It is, therefore, common practice to prescribe an anti-inflammatory agent (most commonly low-dose colchicine 0.5 mg once to twice daily) for 3–6 months after initiating ULT to prevent such flares occurring. Although ULT is not usually commenced during a gout flare for fear of worsening the flare, ULT should not be discontinued if a flare occurs in a patient already taking ULT.

3.8.2   Managing Flares

3.8.2.1 NSAIDs

Despite the nature of the problem being hyperuricaemia for which there is effective treatment, the patient's first need is pain management and for rapid relief of the pain and swelling. All patients experiencing a flare should be advised to use analgesia and to commence its use as early as possible (Finney et al. 2018). The most commonly used drugs to treat gout flares are non-steroidal anti-inflammatory drugs (NSAIDs) (such as Naproxen). NSAIDs should be used at maximum dose due to the severity of pain experienced with a gout flare. It is recommended that NSAIDs are prescribed alongside a gastro protective proton pump inhibitor (PPI) (National Collaborating Centre for Chronic Conditions 2008).

3.8.2.2 Steroids

Oral prednisolone of 30–35 mg daily for 5 days has been shown to be as effective as NSAIDs (Janssens et al. 2008). Expert consensus also suggests that joint aspiration and intra-articular injection of corticosteroids or intramuscular corticosteroid injection are effective treatments (Zhang et al. 2006b).

3.8.2.3 Colchicine

Colchicine is recommended as a first-line treatment for gout alongside NSAIDs. The British National Formulary (BNF) (British National Formulary 2019) recommends the use of colchicine in doses of 0.5 mg two to four times daily. Colchicine may be required for 1–2 weeks in order to prevent rebound flares and can be taken for a further 1–2 days after the flare has subsided (Abhishek et al. 2017). Diarrhoea is a common side effect in the use of colchicine, and for that reason, it should be used cautiously in older patients and in those with CKD (Abhishek et al. 2017). Statins should be stopped while a patient takes colchicine to avoid toxicity (Abhishek et al.

2017). Colchicine can also interact with ciclosporin, ketoconazole, ritonavir, clarithromycin, erythromycin, verapamil and diltiazem among others.

3.9 The British Society of Rheumatology Guideline

The British Society for Rheumatology (BSR) revised their guideline in 2017 (Fig. 3.2). The need for the revision was due to the emergence of new pharmaceutical

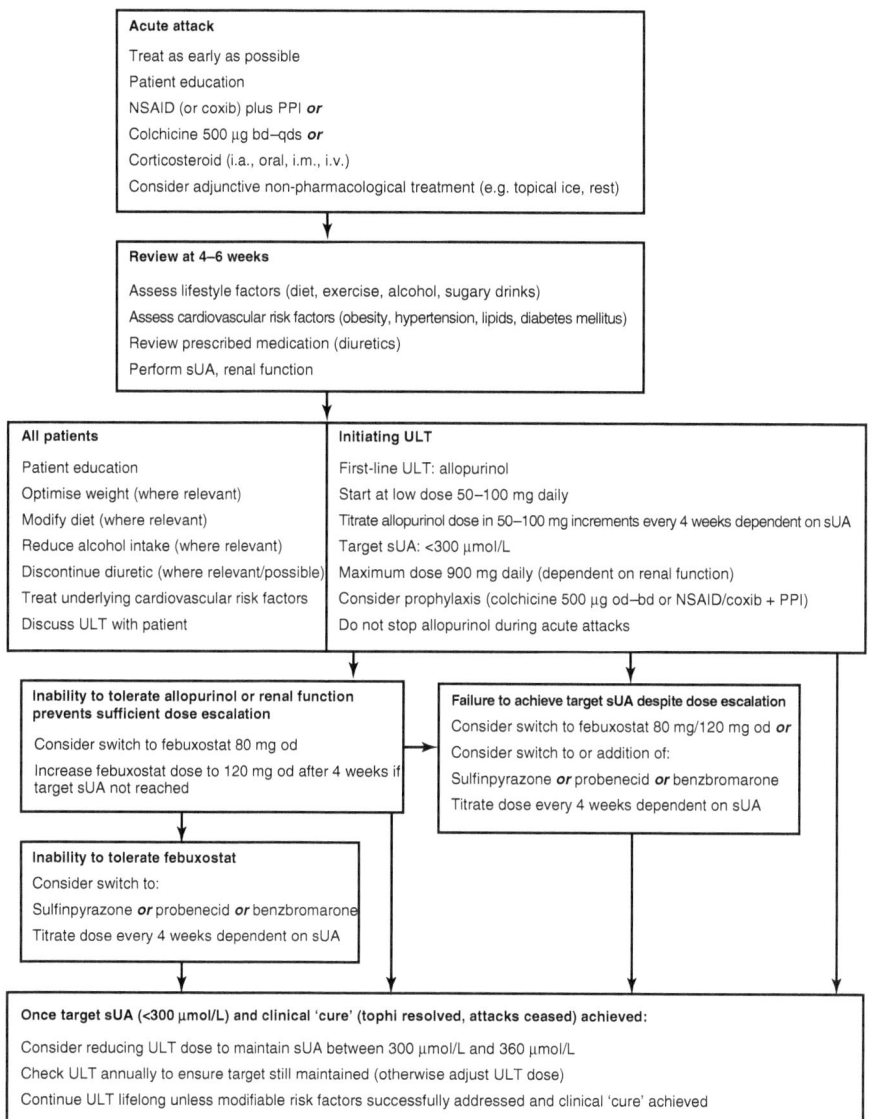

Fig. 3.2 Algorithm for the management of gout. (Source: Hui M, Carr A, Cameron S et al. (2017). The British Society for Rheumatology Guideline for the Management of Gout. *Rheumatology.* 56(7). Reproduced with permission from Rheumatology)

treatment options, the increase in incidence, the prevalence and severity of the condition, the recognised sub-optimal management in both primary and secondary care and a better understanding of the barriers to effective treatment (Hui et al. 2017).

3.9.1 Management of Acute Flares

1. Patients should receive education to better understand acute attacks and how they should be treated. They should be made aware of the importance of continuing their ULT during the attack.
2. The effected joint(s) should be rested, elevated and exposed in a cool environment. A cage over the joint(s) for protection from bed cloths and the use of ice packs can be effective.
3. Maximum dose NSAIDs or Colchicine in doses of 500 μg bd–qds is the drug of choice when there are no contraindications. Patients on NSAIDs or Cox-2 inhibitors should be prescribed gastric protection.
4. Joint aspiration and injection of a corticosteroid are highly effective in acute single joint gout and may be the best treatment in patients with acute illness and comorbidity. A short course of oral corticosteroid or a single injection of an intramuscular corticosteroid is an alternative in patients who are unable to tolerate NSAIDS/colchicine and in whom intra-articular injection is not feasible.
5. In patient with acute gout where response to one treatment is insufficient, combinations of treatment can be used.

3.9.2 Modification of Lifestyle and Risk Factors

1. Where diuretic drugs are being used to treat hypertension rather than heart failure, an alternative anti-hypertensive agent can be considered as long as blood pressure is controlled.
2. All patients with gout should be given verbal and written information about: the causes and consequences of gout and hyperuricaemia; how to manage acute attacks; lifestyle advice about diet, alcohol consumption and obesity; and the use of ULT. Management should be personalised and take into account comorbidities and concurrent medications. Illness perceptions and potential barriers to care should be discussed.
3. Overweight patients should be given dietary modification support to achieve a gradual reduction in body weight, and subsequent maintenance should be encouraged. Diet and exercise should be discussed with all patients, and a well-balanced diet low in fat and added sugars and high in vegetables and fibre should be encouraged: sugar-sweetened soft drinks containing fructose should be avoided, excessive intake of alcoholic drinks and foods high in purine should be avoided. The inclusion of skimmed milk and/or low fat yogurt, soy beans and vegetable sources of protein and cherries should be included in the diet.

4. Gout patients with a history of urolithiasis (bladder stones) should be encouraged to drink more than 2 litres of water daily to avoid dehydration.
5. Patients with cardiovascular (CVD) risk factors and comorbid conditions such as smoking, hypertension, diabetes mellitus, dyslipidaemia, obesity and renal disease should be screened for gout at least annually.

3.9.3 Optimal Use of Urate-Lowering Therapy

1. ULT should be explained to patients when diagnosis is confirmed, and they are being given information about gout. Patients should be fully involved in the decision of when to start ULT. The importance of taking ULT regularly and continually to prevent further attacks should be explained. Patients should be supported during the process of lowering their sUA levels as it can cause an increase in gout flares during this time.
2. ULT should be discussed and offered to all patients who have a diagnosis of gout. ULT should be particularly advised in patients with the following: recurring attacks (>2 attacks in on year); tophi; chronic gouty arthritis; joint damage; renal impairment (eGFR <60 ml/min); a history of urolithiasis; diuretic therapy use and primary gout starting at a young age.
3. Commencement of ULT is best delayed until inflammation has settled as ULT is better discussed when the patient is not in pain.
4. The initial aim of ULT is to reduce and *maintain the sUA level at or below a target level of 300 μmol/l* to prevent further urate crystal formation and to dissolve away existing crystals. The lower the sUA the greater the velocity of crystal elimination. After years of successful treatment, when tophi have resolved and the patient remains free of symptoms, the dose of ULT can be adjusted to maintain the sUA at a level below 300 μmol/l to avoid crystal deposition and the adverse effects of low sUA levels.
5. The recommended first-line ULT is *allopurinol*. It should be started at a low dose (50–100 mg daily), and the dose then increased in 100-mg increments approximately every 4 weeks until the sUA target of *300 μmol/l* has been achieved (maximum dose 900 mg). In patients with renal impairment, small increments (50 mg) should be used and the maximum dose will be lower, but target urate levels should be the same.
6. *Febuxostat* can be used as an alternative second-line XOI for patients in whom allopurinol is not tolerated or whose renal impairment prevents allopurinol dose escalation sufficient to achieve the therapeutic target. Start with a dose of 80 mg daily and if necessary increase after 4 weeks to 120 mg daily to achieve therapeutic target.
7. Uricosuric agents can be used in patients who are resistant to, or intolerant of, XOIs. The preferred drugs are sulfinpyrazone (200–800 mg/day) or probenecid (500–2000 mg/day) in patients with normal or mildly impaired renal function or benzbromarone (50–200 mg/day) in patients with mild-to-moderate renal insufficiency.

8. Losartan and fenofibrate should not be used as a primary ULT, but where treatment for hypertension or dyslipidaemia, respectively, is required, they may be considered as they have a weak uricosuric effect. Vitamin C supplements (500–1500 mg daily) also have a weak uricosuric effect.
9. A uricosuric agent can be used in combination with XOIs in patients who do not achieve a therapeutic serum urate target with optimal doses on monotherapy.
10. Colchicine 500 μg bd or od should be considered as a prophylaxis against acute attacks resulting from initiation or up-titration of any ULT and continued for up to 6 months. In patients who cannot tolerate colchicine, a low-dose NSAID or coxib, with gastro-protection, can be used as an alternative, providing there are no contraindications.

The full British Society Rheumatology Guideline is available at *Rheumatology* online.

3.10 The Role for the Healthcare Professional

The high prevalence of gout means that it is most frequently treated by GPs, with only the most difficult of cases referred to secondary care rheumatologists (Abhishek and Doherty 2018). Many primary care healthcare professionals have significant gaps in their knowledge, and they may have inaccurate views of the pathogenesis of gout, have over-emphasis of the importance of lifestyle factors and be unaware of cut-off levels for hyperuricaemia and target levels for sUA (Abhishek and Doherty 2018). Primary care GPs and nurses put this lack of knowledge down to inadequate knowledge and insufficient training around gout (Spencer et al. 2012; Vaccher et al. 2016).

Equally, patients with gout also have a gap in their knowledge and understanding of the condition that affects them. Patient education is vital in the management of gout in order to get patients to commence on the right medication and to improve the long-term adherence to that medication. Only 30–40% of patients with gout receive ULT, 30–40% of those receive sub-optimal doses and adherence to ULT is less than 40% at 12 months (Abhishek et al. 2017).

A well-informed nurse who has a good understanding of gout and its treatment and management is essential to improve patient understanding and self-management. It is also important to be able to signpost patients to the best written information or websites. The United Kingdom patient charity, Versus Arthritis offer both written information and a dedicated website (https://www.versusarthritis.org/about-arthritis/conditions/gout/) to help those with gout. Furthermore, nurses can direct patients to the 'healthtalk.org' website. This website (http://www.healthtalk.org/peoples-experiences/bones-joints/gout/topics) has an extensive section covering gout with videos from health professionals who treat gout and people who are living with gout.

A trial by Doherty and colleagues (Doherty et al. 2018) showed that primary care nurse-led gout management brings about significant clinical improvements and achieves treat-to-target gout recommendations. Their intervention, involving high-quality patient education, managing gout as a long-term condition and treatment escalation using a clear protocol demonstrated that nurses can make significant improvements for gout outcomes. Secondary care rheumatology nurses are not currently involved in the care of patients with gout universally, but the results of the Doherty trial raise the possibility that rheumatology nurses can make a huge contribution to improve the care of this prevalent but frequently poorly managed condition.

Summary of Main Points
1. A combination of pharmacological (NSAIDS and colchicine) and non-pharmacological (ice packs) interventions can be used to reduce the pain in acute gout attacks.
2. ULT correctly titrated is the gold standard treatment and will reduce and resolve acute gout attacks in the long term.
3. ULT should be titrated (treat to target) until the target of 300 µmol/l is reached.
4. Those with gout should receive guidance and education on the condition to gain a better understanding.
5. Nurses and other healthcare professionals (HCPs) need to support patients with lifestyle advice and supported self-management.
6. To improve current sub-optimal management, nurses and other HCPs should be guided by the BSR (2017) Gout recommendations.

3.11 Self-Assessment

Assessing your own learning having read the chapter, the following are some ideas as to how to relate what you have learnt to your practice

1. Consider what you currently know about gout having read this chapter. Try explaining gout to a colleague to gauge your understanding and ability to transfer this knowledge to staff and patients.
2. Discuss with your colleagues the most effective drug treatments to use in gout (discuss pain management, prophylaxis and ULT).
3. Discuss with your colleagues the lifestyle adaptations patients can make to reduce the chances of gout flare.

References

Abhishek, Doherty. Education and non-pharmacological approaches for gout. Rheumatology. 2018;57:i57–8.

Abhishek A, Roddy E, Doherty M. Gout—a guide for the general and acute physicians. Clin Med (Lond). 2017;17(1):54–9.

Becker MA, Schumacher HR Jr, Wortmann RE, et al. Febuxostat compared with allopurinol in patients with hyperuricemia and gout. N Engl J Med. 2005;353(23):2450–61.

British National Formulary. Colchicine. 2019. https://bnf.nice.org.uk/drug/colchicine.html. Accessed 02.05.19.

Bucknall M, Mallen C, Muller S, Hayward R, West S, Choi H, Roddy E. Gout as a consequence of obstructive sleep apnoea: a matched cohort study. Arthritis Rheum. 2018 Aug 30; https://doi.org/10.1002/art.40662.

Bursill D, Taylor WJ, Terkeltaub R, et al. Gout, hyperuricemia, and crystal-associated disease network consensus statement regarding labels and definitions for disease elements in gout. Arthritis Care Res. 2019;71(13):427–34.

Dalbeth N, Merriman TR, Stamp LK. Gout. Lancet. 2016;388:2019–52.

Doherty M, Jenkins W, Richardson H, et al. Efficacy and cost-effectiveness of nurse-led care involving education and engagement of patients and a treat-to-target urate-lowering strategy versus usual care for gout: a randomised controlled trial. Lancet. 2018;392(10156):1403–12.

Finney AG, Viggars R, Roddy E. Gout: Is there a role in management for the general practice nurse? Pract Nurse. 2018 Aug 18:23–5.

Hui M, Carr A, Cameron S, et al. The British Society for Rheumatology Guideline for the Management of Gout. Rheumatology (Oxford). 2017;56(7):e1–e20.

Janssens HJ, Janssen M, van de Lisdonk, et al. Use of oral prednisolone or naproxen for the treatment of gout arthritis: a double-blind, randomised equivalence trial. Lancet. 2008;371(9627):1854–60.

Kuo CF, Grainge MG, Mallen CD, et al. Rising burden of gout in the UK but continuing suboptimal management: a nationwide population study. Ann Rheum Dis. 2015;74:661–7.

National Collaborating Centre for Chronic Conditions. Osteoarthritis Clinical Guideline for care and management in adults. London: Royal College of Physicians; 2008.

Punzi L. Change gout: the need for a new approach. Minerva Med. 2017;108(4):341–9.

Rees F, Doherty M. Patients with gout can be cured in primary care. Practitioner. 2014;258(1777):15–9.

Rees F, Hui M, Doherty M. Optimising current treatment of gout. Nat Rev Rheumatol. 2014;10(5):271–83.

Richardson JC, Liddle J, Mallen CD, et al. A joint effort over a period of time: factors affecting use of urate-lowering therapy for long-term treatment of gout. BMC Musculoskeletal Disorder. 2016;17:249.

Roddy E, Choi HK. Epidemiology of gout. Rheum Dis Clin North Am. 2014;40(2):155–75.

Roddy E, Mallen CD, Doherty M. Clinical review: gout. BMJ. 2013;347:f5648.

Spencer K, Carr A, Doherty M. Patient and provider barriers to effective management of gout in in general practice: a qualitative study. Ann Rheum Dis. 2012;71:1490–5.

Vaccher S, Kannangara DR, Baysari MT, et al. Barriers to care in gout: from prescriber to patient. J Rheumatol. 2016;43:144–9.

Versus Arthritis. Gout. 2019. https://www.versusarthritis.org/about-arthritis/conditions/gout/. Accessed 02.05.19.

Zhang W, Doherty M, Pascual E, Bardin T, Barskova, et al. EULAR Standing Committee for International Clinical Studies Including Therapeutics. EULAR evidence based recommendations for gout. Part 1: Diagnosis. Report of a task force of the Standing Committee for International Clinical Studies Including Therapeutics (ESCISIT). Ann Rheum Dis. 2006a;65:1301–11.

Zhang W, Doherty M, Pascual E, Bardin T, Barskova, et al. EULAR Standing Committee for International Clinical Studies Including Therapeutics. EULAR evidence based recommendations for gout. Part 2: Management. Report of a task force of the Standing Committee for International Clinical Studies Including Therapeutics (ESCISIT). Ann Rheum Dis. 2006b;65:1312–24.

Zhu Y, Pandya B, Choi H. Comorbidities of gout and hyperuricemia in the US general population: NHANES 2077–2008. Am J Med. 2012;125:679687.

Further Reading

https://www.goutstudygroup.com/patients/ is a useful resource for patients to learn more about gout.

Polymyalgia Rheumatica

4

Anne O'Brien

4.1 Learning Outcomes

Having read this chapter and following further study, the reader will be able to:

1. Recognise a patient presenting with possible PMR and GCA.
2. Provide some initial patient education and symptom management advice.
3. Describe a typical care pathway for a patient with PMR.
4. Identify which health professionals are most appropriate to support and manage patients with PMR.

4.2 Introduction to PMR

Polymyalgia rheumatica is one of the commonest inflammatory rheumatic disorders affecting older people typically over the age of 70. Originally thought to be a form of gout (Bruce 1888), PMR was first proposed as a discrete condition in 1957 (Barber 1957).

Many consider it difficult to diagnose because the classic signs and symptoms mimic other musculoskeletal and rheumatological conditions (Mackie and Mallen 2013). However, key features include sudden onset of bilateral shoulder and pelvic girdle muscle pain and stiffness, without small joint inflammation.

PMR can disrupt and significantly impact on an individual's day-to-day functioning and quality of life (Dejaco et al. 2015), but usually has a good prognosis, with most people not requiring medical management after 5 years.

A. O'Brien (✉)

School of Primary, Community and Social Care, Keele University, Newcastle, UK

e-mail: a.v.o'brien@keele.ac.uk

© Springer Nature Switzerland AG 2020

S. Ryan (ed.), *Nursing Older People with Arthritis and other Rheumatological Conditions*, Perspectives in Nursing Management and Care for Older Adults, https://doi.org/10.1007/978-3-030-18012-6_4

45

This chapter presents the latest evidence relating to PMR management to enable the nurse to identify patients with PMR as early as possible.

4.2.1 PMR and Giant Cell Arteritis (GCA)

PMR is associated with giant cell arteritis (GCA) (Petri et al. 2015), an inflammation of the arteries affecting the neck and head. This is the most common form of large-/medium-vessel vasculitis. Approximately one in five patients with PMR also have GCA, while 40–60% of people with GCA have PMR symptoms at diagnosis (Salvarani et al. 2008). Undiagnosed, untreated GCA may lead to serious consequences, including potential permanent sight loss. Nurses can play a vital role in early recognition of the features of both PMR and GCA (Leslie et al. 2003).

4.3 Aetiology

The cause of PMR is not yet fully understood (Mackie and Mallen 2013), although some suggest that there may be both environmental and genetic predisposing factors (Kermani and Warrington 2013), although genetic links are, as yet, unproven. An association with the HLA-DRB1∗04 gene has been observed in people originally from northern, but not southern, Europe (Gonzalez-Gay et al. 2009). Links to infective agents have also been hypothesised, but they are also yet to be demonstrated (Kermani and Warrington 2013; Gonzalez-Gay et al. 2009). Other theories include a possible age-related decline in the hypothalamic–pituitary–gonadal axis resulting in adrenal insufficiency (Straub and Cutolo 2006), but a definitive cause is yet to be established.

4.4 Pathogenesis

Also lacking in consensus is the pathogenesis of PMR, although histological studies confirm an inflammatory element probably giving origin to the classic neck and pelvic aching symptoms. Inflammation is observed on MRI and ultrasound imaging (Kermani and Warrington 2013) as periarticular synovitis (inflammation of the synovium around joints), bursitis and tenosynovitis (Dasgupta 2013) or shoulder or hip effusions (increased amounts of synovial fluid) (Frediani et al. 2002).

Synovitis has also been identified from histological scrutiny of shoulder biopsies where macrophages and CD4 T cells have been identified (Kreiner et al. 2010). Some suggest the oedema within the synovial sheaths of tendons, rather than synovial hyperplasia (the production of more synovial cells) is the more likely origin of pain and stiffness symptoms in PMR (Falsetti et al. 2011).

The role of inflammatory mediators is yet to be fully understood. Elevated interleukin (IL)-6 levels are seen in both PMR and GCA, and raised IL 1-1β is also observed in PMR patients (Alvarez-Rodríguez et al. 2010), both of which are thought to potentially explain some of the systemic features of the condition (Kreiner et al. 2010).

4.5   Incidence and Prevalence

The lifetime reported risk is 2.4% for females and 1.7% for males (Crowson et al. 2011). PMR is more prevalent in women (affecting two to three times more women than men) and much more likely to be observed in older adults (Salvarani et al. 2008; Smeeth et al. 2006).

The incidence of new diagnoses in PMR appears to be slightly increasing (Raheel et al. 2017), potentially explained by ageing populations, especially as the mean age of PMR onset is reported to be 73 years (Kermani and Warrington 2013). Geography also appears to influence incidence, higher incidence being observed for people living in the northern hemisphere, increasing with northern latitudes residence (Gonzalez-Gay et al. 2009). Norway has reported the highest incidence of 112.6 per 100,000 population per year over the age of 50 (Gran and Myklebust 1997), while UK statistics also suggest a slightly increasing incidence rate observed over a 10-year period, averaging at 84 (Smeeth et al. 2006) to 96 (Partington et al. 2018a) new diagnoses of PMR per 100,000 population per year.

The overall prevalence of PMR in a population over the age of 50 is thought to be between 0.1% and 1% (Hayward et al. 2014; Salvarani et al. 1995). A prevalence rate for women over the age of 50 has been reported in the United States to be 870 and 508 in males per 100,000 population (Crowson and Matteson 2017), although UK data suggest a higher combined gender prevalence of 1000 per 100,000 (Hayward et al. 2014).

4.6   Clinical Presentation: Signs and Symptoms

A typical history will include reported bilateral shoulder pain referring into the upper arms, often described as an ache, developing within a few days, with no obvious cause. This rapid onset of upper limb pain is important, as this is the most commonly presenting and documented PMR symptom reported in primary care settings (Helliwell et al. 2013) and differentiates many patients from osteoarthritis symptoms, which typically progress over months. PMR-related pains tend to exacerbated by activity and disturb sleep (Salvarani et al. 2008). Initial symptoms are often reported to be preceded by fatigue impacting on daily life (Green et al. 2015), general malaise and sometimes fever.

Typically more a muscle (than joint) pain, patients often experience tenderness on palpation of larger muscle groups around the shoulders and (less commonly) the pelvic girdle which is often accompanied by enduring stiffness, lasting possibly hours into the day and sometimes night (Twohig et al. 2015; Muller et al. 2016). Many patients report great reluctance to move for fear of exacerbating the pain. Hip pain (which may refer into the upper thighs) and neck ache are also reported in

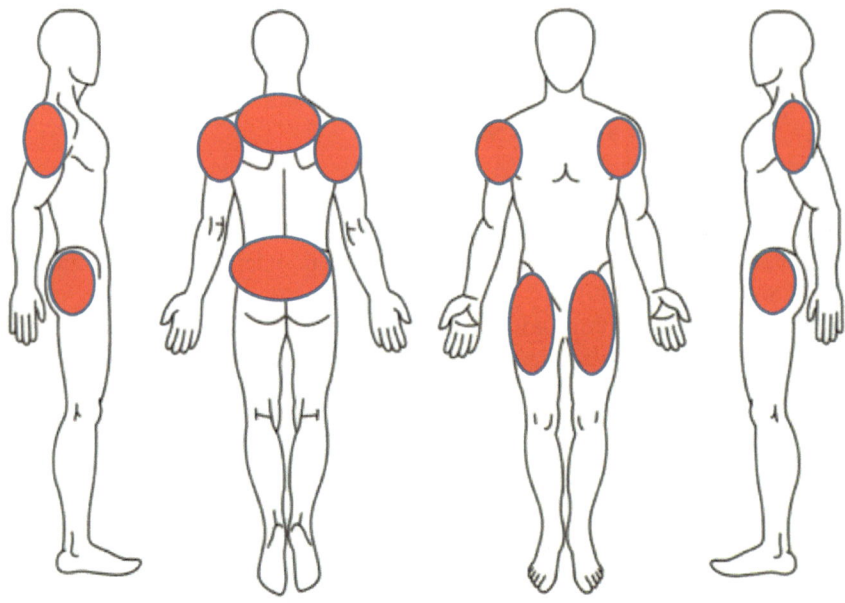

Fig. 4.1 Illustrating typical anatomical areas affected in PMR. Key: (⬤) Distribution of typically described pain/ache/stiffness in PMR

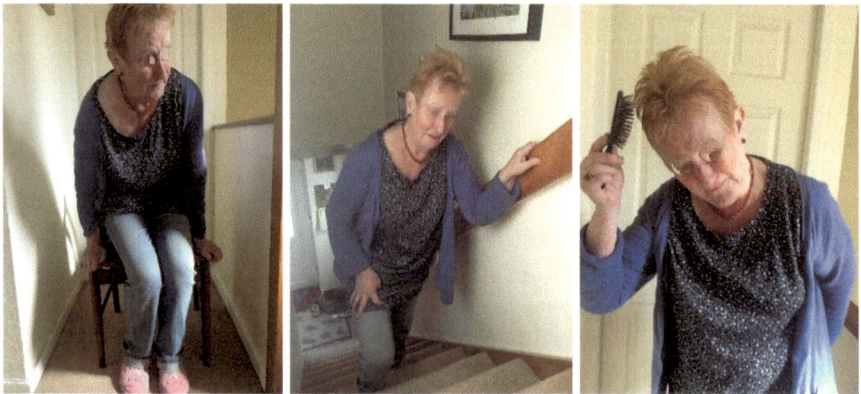

Fig. 4.2 Illustrating challenging activities of daily living for the patient with PMR. (Copyright and courtesy of B Jessop 2019)

50–70% of people first presenting with PMR. Figure 4.1 shows the typical anatomical sites affected in PMR.

A newly diagnosed PMR patient may typically report a sudden onset and difficulty, undertaking everyday life activities, such as getting out of a chair, climbing stairs, getting dressed or lifting objects, especially anything requiring overhead movement (Fig. 4.2).

While many patients also report feeling weak, this is usually due to reduced activity, secondary to pain. Objectively measurable weakness is not, however, a primary feature of PMR (although may later be a consequence of taking long-term glucocorticoids) so may, at initial presentation, cause clinicians to question the diagnosis. All these challenges impact on an individual's ability to move freely in everyday life as well as quality of life (Dejaco et al. 2015; Mackie et al. 2014).

Some patients may also present with other systemic features, such as malaise, low-grade fever, depression, loss of appetite or weight loss, which has been reported to occur in up to 40% of people with PMR (Salvarani et al. 1987). Relapse of symptoms is unfortunately common. Mindful of the serious consequences of a missed diagnosis, nurses and all health professionals should always consider if a patient with PMR might also have GCA.

4.6.1 Clinical Presentation in GCA

- Headaches or occipital tenderness
- Scalp or temporal tenderness—noticed when combing their hair or putting on headwear
- Jaw pain or tongue ache—noticeable when chewing
- Unusual sensory changes in limbs or peripheral claudication symptoms, absent pulses
- Ear pain
- Intermittent eyesight disturbance
- Cough, hoarseness or a sore throat
- Carotidynia, an inflammation of the carotid artery—throbbing pain of the neck and face

Any of these symptoms should be noted as potential 'GCA red flags', and nurses strongly suspecting GCA should refer patients for urgent specialist advice or advise patients to seek emergency medical attention to avoid the risk of permanent sight damage (Kermani and Warrington 2013).

4.7 Diagnosis

Despite first being described in 1888, there is still no gold standard diagnostic test for PMR. It is generally agreed, however, that diagnosis should only be proposed following a clinical examination and identifying elevated inflammatory markers; typically both the erythrocyte sedimentation rate (ESR) and C-reactive protein (CRP) levels are raised in the blood (Kermani and Warrington 2013; Seitz 2015).

Diagnosis can be challenging (Mackie and Pease 2013), largely because symptoms may be somewhat vague, could be accounted for by several other diagnoses, but also may originate from other comorbidities, for example, osteoarthritis (OA), commonly seen in older people or as a result of polypharmacy issues, for example, statin-induced muscle aches. Consequently, careful investigation is important to try to avoid errors in provisional diagnoses (Table 4.1).

Table 4.1 Clinical symptoms, differential diagnoses and relevant investigations in PMR

Symptom on clinical presentation	Differential diagnoses	Related relevant investigations	Comment
Shoulder girdle pain	Rheumatoid arthritis	Anti-CCP Rheumatoid factor Ultrasound	RA likely to have wrist and finger synovitis
	Septic arthritis	Hand/foot X-ray Inflammatory markers; ESR, CRP	Erosions on X-ray Raised inflammatory marker
	Rotator cuff disorders[a] Shoulder impingement[a] Adhesive capsulitis (frozen shoulder)[a]		Normal inflammatory markers Restriction and pain on shoulder abduction, internal and external rotations
Hip girdle pain	Osteoarthritis hip	Plain film X-ray	Narrowing of joint margins; reduced hip rotation
	Trochanteric bursitis[a]		Tenderness lateral hip
Neck and back pain	Spondyloarthropathy Cervical or lumbar spondylosis Ankylosing spondylitis/Sacroiliitis	Plain film X-ray Inflammatory markers; ESR, CRP	Observe degenerative changes, facet joints Normal inflammatory markers
	Giant cell arteritis	Temporal artery biopsy, inflammatory markers, ESR, CRP	Raised inflammatory markers
	Myeloma	Immunoglobulins, protein electrophoresis, Bence–Jones urine test	
	Spinal osteoporosis (vertebral wedge fracture)	DEXA scan	
Stiffness lasting > 30 min	Inflammatory condition, e.g. RA; connective tissue disorders, e.g. SLE, vasculitis, systemic sclerosis	Inflammatory markers, ESR, CRP Auto-antibodies	Raised inflammatory markers
Reported limb weakness	Polymyositis	CK levels	If proximal weakness with little/no pain
	RA Carpal tunnel	Inflammatory markers, ESR, CRP	

Table 4.1 (continued)

Symptom on clinical presentation	Differential diagnoses	Related relevant investigations	Comment
Fatigue	Fibromyalgia	FBC	Normal inflammatory markers
	Thyroid dysfunction	Thyroid-stimulating hormone (TSH)	Abnormal TSH levels
	Malignancy Infection, e.g. UTI	Screening CXR	Raised white cell count
Fever	Osteomyelitis Endocarditis	FBC, infection screen, glucose, U&E	

Informed by Kermani and Warrington (2013) and Hennell et al. (2007)). Also see Investigations: Section 4.8.1

Key: *Anti-CCP* anti-cyclic citrullinated peptide, *ESR* erythrocyte sedimentation rate, *CRP* C-reactive protein, *CK* creatinine phosphokinase, *FBC* full blood count, *CXR* chest X-ray, *RA* rheumatoid arthritis, *OA* osteoarthritis, *TSH* thyroid-stimulating hormone, *DEXA* dual-energy X-ray absorptiometry, *U&E* urea and electrolytes, *UTI* urinary tract infection, *SLE* systemic lupus erythematosus

[a]More likely to be unilateral

The required clinical criteria to apply the scoring algorithm include: age >50 years, bilateral shoulder aching and abnormal C reactive protein. If these clinical criteria are present then the following point system can be applied as stated below:

1) Morning stiffness (duration >45 minutes)   (2 points)
2) Hip pain or limited range of motion (1 point)
3) Absence of rheumatoid factor or anti-cyclic citrullinated peptide antibodies (2 points)
4) Absence of other joint pain (1 point)
5) On ultrasound scan at least one abnormal shoulder and at least one abnormal hip (1 point)
6) On ultrasound scan both shoulders abnormal (1 point)

A score ≥4, patient is categorised as PMR without ultrasound and a score of 5 or more is categorised as PMR with ultrasound

Fig. 4.3 The 2012 EULAR/ACR scoring algorithm for classification criteria of polymyalgia rheumatica (Dasgupta et al. 2012a)

Current guidelines for the management of PMR recommend that key pathologies should be excluded before a safe and confident diagnosis of PMR be given (Dejaco et al. 2015), in particular, rheumatoid arthritis (RA), active infection or cancer (De Bandt 2014). This appears to be particularly important in the first 6 months of presentation when incidence rate of new cancers is higher (Muller et al. 2014).

The 2012 EULAR/ARC scoring algorithm for the classification criteria of PMR is reported to have a high sensitivity (92.6%) and specificity (91.3%), with ultrasound included, reduced to 81.5% without ultrasound (Macchioni et al. 2014) (Fig. 4.3).

Using these internationally agreed criteria, endorsed by both the European League Against Rheumatism (EULAR) (Dasgupta et al. 2012a) and the American College of Rheumatology (Dasgupta et al. 2012b), should improve the consistency of PMR classification and, in particular, the likelihood of successfully differentiating PMR from early-onset RA. However, as originally developed for clinical trial purposes, these classification criteria are not intended to be used as diagnostic criteria (Mackie and Mallen 2013).

In light of the close association with GCA, any patient suspected to have PMR should also be examined to exclude GCA.

4.8 Investigations

To optimise diagnostic accuracy and speed, it is important to actively exclude other possible causes of PMR symptoms, particularly an inflammatory arthritis, infection or malignancy (Table 4.1). The British Society of Rheumatology, therefore, advocates a range of screening investigations starting with blood tests to help confirm PMR and exclude other diagnoses (Dasgupta et al. 2010; Owen et al. 2015).

4.8.1 Blood Tests

Bloods tests, urinalysis, chest X-ray and ultrasonography should be completed before a PMR diagnosis is confirmed (Brown et al. 2014).

- *Erythrocyte sedimentation rate (ESR) and C-reactive protein (CRP)* are the most commonly requested inflammatory marker blood tests for both diagnostic and monitoring purposes.
  - While the CRP may be more sensitive, both are likely to be raised in untreated PMR (and GCA).
  - The ESR is usually raised and may even exceed 100 mm/h, although in a small proportion of patients (thought to be up to 1 in 5), the ESR may be within normal limits (Kermani and Warrington 2013).
  - Both the ESR and CRP are assessed over time with reducing levels, suggesting treatment efficacy and improvement.
  - Raised markers should be cautiously interpreted and infection or an inflammatory arthritis also considered as possible causes.
- *A full blood count* (FBC) helps to exclude infection and anaemia; checking for normochromic normocytic anaemia is recommended if patients appear pale.
- *Urea and electrolytes* will evaluate renal function.
- *The thyroid-stimulating hormone (TSH)* blood test can and should easily be assessed to exclude thyroid dysfunction especially if fatigue, malaise and lethargy are prominent reported symptoms. Clinicians should also remember, however, that TSH levels normally increase with age.

- *Dipstick urinalysis* is also valuable to help quickly exclude infection and other mimicking conditions. If malignancy is suspected, a protein electrophoresis over a 24-hour urine collection may be advisable. The absence of the Bence–Jones protein helps to rule out multiple myeloma, more commonly seen in people over the age of 60.
- *Additional blood tests* which should be negative in PMR, but can help to exclude other pathologies are (Kermani and Warrington 2013) as follows:
  - Rheumatoid factor—positive in RA.
  - Anti-cyclic citrullinated peptide (anti-CCP)—raised in RA.
  - Anti-nuclear antibodies—positive in systemic auto-immune conditions, for example, SLE, infections or some cancers.
  - Creatinine phosphokinase (CPK)—raised in myositis or myopathy.
  - Alanine and aspartate transaminase (ALT and AST)—indicate liver pathology.

4.8.2 Imaging

Ultrasound (US) imaging is not routine, but may be particularly useful to differentiate between inconclusive bilateral shoulder symptoms (Sakellariou et al. 2013), particularly elderly onset RA, spondyloarthritis or calcium pyrophosphate deposition disease (Falsetti et al. 2011), as well as playing a role in classifying PMR.

Magnetic resonance imaging (MRI) additionally plays a role evidencing shoulder sub-acromial bursitis, tenosynovitis or hip trochanteric bursitis that may accompany a PMR presentation and slightly enhances the specificity and sensitivity of a PMR diagnosis. However, if glenohumeral synovitis is observed, a diagnosis of RA is more likely than PMR (Ruta et al. 2012).

In complex presentations, occasionally positron emission tomography (PET) scans may be used to either illustrate extra-articular synovial structures around the hips, shoulders or neck, to support a diagnosis if symptoms are perplexing, or identify a vasculitis if GCA is suspected, as uptake may be observed in vessels, for example, in sub-clavian arteries (Kermani and Warrington 2013).

4.8.3 GCA Investigations

Patients with probable PMR should be questioned explicitly about possible GCA symptoms (see Section 4.6.1), and where GCA is suspected, peripheral pulses should be examined. Subsequent investigations may include ultrasound imaging (particularly to evaluate inflammation in potentially 'silent' anatomical areas such as the aorta (Salvarani et al. 2013)); a temporal artery biopsy, which if positive confirms a GCA diagnosis; and/or referral for an ophthalmology opinion.

4.9   Medical Management

Physician's role: General practitioners diagnose and manage approximately 70% of PMR patients in primary care settings (Yates et al. 2016). The physician's first role is to confirm a PMR diagnosis by excluding other pathologies via thorough history taking and basic laboratory testing, including the ESR and CRP inflammatory markers which help support the PMR diagnosis (see Sections 4.7 and 4.8). More complex patients, typically younger patients, those with inconclusive diagnoses, who are not responding to early treatment or have concurrent comorbidities, may be referred to seek specialist advice, often from a rheumatologist. Nurses can also, however, play an invaluable role listening to, counselling and educating patients at this early stage of diagnosis.

Glucocorticoid therapy: PMR management guidelines agreed internationally largely focus upon the early introduction of glucocorticoid (steroid) therapy, usually administered orally with prednisolone. A glucocorticoid (GC) starting dose may typically be 12.5–25 mg/day and is calculated from an individual's weight, not perception of symptom severity, with 15 mg being a recommended starting dose for the first 3 weeks for patients presenting with probable diagnoses of PMR (Dejaco et al. 2015). Improvement in PMR symptoms can be dramatic within 72 hours and helps reassure clinicians of diagnosis. Steroid dosage should then be reduced to 10 mg/day within 1–2 months, which if remission is sustained, can be further reduced by 1 mg per month until asymptomatic.

A minimum of 12 months GC treatment is expected, although gradual tapering over a period of years without recurrence of symptoms is more common. Patients with intransigent, or relapsing PMR, may also require supplementary steroid sparing agents such as methotrexate or azathioprine. For many patients (around 25%), GCs are needed to manage symptoms for over 4 years (Partington et al. 2018b) and possibly as many as 6 years (Shbeeb et al. 2018).

Monitoring: While on steroid therapy, ongoing monitoring is important and may be part of the nursing role. Having a moderate correlation with the Health Assessment Questionnaire (HAQ) (Fries et al. 1980) (a patient-reported questionnaire evaluating disability and function) captures some of the everyday functional items important to PMR patients (Mackie et al. 2014). Additionally, the serial monitoring of C-reactive protein is probably the most valuable measure of disease activity, which guides patient management in day-to-day clinical practice (Helliwell et al. 2016).

Adverse events: Unfortunately, however, despite a usually positive reduction in symptoms, up to 50% of people with PMR experience adverse events associated with GC therapy (Salvarani et al. 2008), some of which may be life threatening (Fardet 2013). Consequently, direct and rapid access for patients to medical advice is, therefore, also a strong recommendation from the international guidelines (Dejaco et al. 2015).

Informed patients, aware of significant associated adverse events, may, therefore, not only be reluctant to start taking GCs but also very keen to stop taking them as soon as possible (Muller et al. 2018). The nurse will, therefore, have a very important educational and supportive role reinforcing the rationale for and promoting

Table 4.2 Adverse events associated with glucocorticoid therapy in PMR

• Osteoporosis (and fragility fracture risk) (Paskins et al. 2018)
• Mood changes, depression (Vivekanantham et al. 2018)
• Increased risk of infection
• Bruising/fragility of the skin
• Increased risk of cardiovascular disease/events (Partington et al. 2018a; Fardet and Fève 2014)
• Weight gain
• Uncontrolled hypertension
• Diabetes
• Glaucoma
• Muscle weakness (myopathy)
• Adrenal insufficiency

Informed by Fardet and Fève (2014), Partington et al. (2018a), Paskins et al. (2018), and Vivekanantham et al. (2018)

concordance with the GC prescription. Once started, the dose has to be carefully balanced to achieve symptom reduction, while also minimising the cumulative dose to reduce the risk of developing any of the known associated side effects and complications (Table 4.2).

The osteoporosis (OP) and fragility fracture risk is possibly one of the most well-known side effects, with associated significant morbidity in older patients. Studies suggest an increased overall fracture risk (63%) in PMR compared to population controls (Paskins et al. 2018) with the risk of bone loss greatest in the first 3 months and risk of fracture increases by as much as 75% following commencement of GC therapy (Van Staa et al. 2003). This concurrent and rapid decrease in bone mineral density may be as much as 6–12% within the first 12 months, and consequently, clinicians will try to reduce the steroid dose as quickly as possible.

Nurses can help identify those most at risk, ordering a dual-energy X-ray absorptiometry (DXA) scan at this stage may be useful to gain baseline measures of bone density. Additionally, bisphosphonates may be prescribed to further reduce fracture risk (Hennell 2004) with nurses playing important educational and drug counselling roles.

4.10 The Nursing Assessment

A holistic and open-minded approach is central to the assessment of a patient with PMR (Whitlock and Hollywood 2014). Nurses working in advanced practice roles may be the first to consider a PMR diagnosis, so previous discussion around clinical presentation and diagnosis will be relevant and contribute to their early assessments.

PMR or MSK symptoms: Discerning whether patients have symptoms originating from underlying musculoskeletal (MSK) or inflammatory conditions is, however, a skilful aspect of all nurses' roles, so familiarity with and knowledge of other prevalent MSK conditions, especially OA and RA, will be important. However, for most nurses encountering patients with a confirmed primary or comorbid PMR diagnosis, symptom reduction and patient education will be the management focus. There may also be changes to the musculoskeletal system related to ageing including the gradual loss of muscle mass and strength (referred to as sarcopenia), which may negatively impact on function.

Evaluating patient fears: Depending on the timing of a nursing assessment post diagnosis, patients may well be uncertain about the PMR condition; the majority are likely to have never heard of PMR before this health episode (Muller et al. 2018). Consequently, many may appear fearful of the impact of this diagnosis on their lives and may be reluctant to start GC medication. Allowing time with patients, therefore, will be important to gain understanding of their knowledge of the condition, listen to and address their specific concerns and educate them further about PMR and the support available to them.

Establishing patient knowledge: A significant aspect of the assessment will include an evaluation of the patient's knowledge and understanding of prescribed glucocorticoid medication and 'red flag' monitoring signs. Does the patient understand, for example:

- The rationale behind medication dosage
- Possible adverse effects to observe for
- Relevance of blood test results
- Symptoms and signs which may suggest deterioration
- How to act upon any GCA symptoms
- Who to contact if they have additional concerns

Some nurses may have access to steroid treatment cards to offer patients. Sometimes also given by pharmacists, these cards allow patients to alert others to their prescription as well as facilitating patients to record their cumulative dose over time. Issuing a steroid card to an older person may help cognitive ability as short-term memory declines gradually over time.

Compliance with medication: The nurse is especially well placed to evaluate the patient's likely compliance with medication (Hennell 2004). Part of their assessment can, therefore, involve discussion about the patient's general medical history (and concordance with medical management) as well as their most recent health story, which should include how PMR symptoms are impacting on daily life.

Activities of daily living: General physical independence levels may be assessed and can be observed from the first encounter as a patient approaches a consultation room. This may include an overall evaluation of mobility, the support offered (+/− accepted) by accompanying family/friend, as well as observing how the individual sits down or removes clothing. Often with older patients, there can be a decline in function due to alterations in muscle tone and the patient may need advice in exercises to increase muscle strength. If a physical examination is required, skin condition and any obvious muscle wastage can also be gauged. It may also be at such a time that other features may be observed, for example, significant synovitis, in which case, the nurse may reflect on the diagnosis; might the patient be presenting as a PMR onset of RA where pitting oedema of hands or feet tenosynovitis? (Hennell et al. 2007).

Therapist referrals: The nurse will determine if referral for rehabilitation and specific patient education relating to activities of daily living (washing, dressing, mobility and driving) may be appropriate. Physiotherapy referrals may focus on symptom management but will also promote physical activity and functional independence using exercise therapy and will involve considering the effects of ageing on movement and balance. Occupational therapy referrals may request additional home assessments to promote maintaining normal life.

Psychological support: The nurse may also establish that some patients appearing distressed or fearful may need additional psychological support. This may be particularly noticeable in patients who have had delayed diagnoses, those who have had significant changes in lifestyle since the sudden onset of symptoms (Kennedy-Malone and Enevold 2001) or those who may have suspected malignancy prior to their PMR diagnosis. In older people, depression is often associated with other illnesses and often under treated.

4.11 The Nurses Role in Management of PMR

4.11.1 Holistic Management Approach

The nurse may be key to co-ordinating a holistic approach to patient management in PMR and fulfil a monitoring and educational role. The nurse is well placed to routinely include some of the outcome measures, which are varied and numerous in PMR, but will typically include some measurement of pain, stiffness and global assessment identified by both the patient and clinician in addition to inflammatory markers (Duarte et al. 2015).

Each consultation should allow patients to report their lived experience with PMR and will lead the nurse to decide what subsequent monitoring is needed. This may specifically include an evaluation of:

- Inflammatory markers—ESR, CRP
- The reason for persistent symptoms; pain, stiffness, fatigue—numerical rating scales
- Impact on daily life—Health Anxiety Questionnaire (HAQ)
- Psychological health—Hospital Anxiety and Depression (HAD) Scale

Nurses may be one of the first health professionals to identify the patient's need for psychological support (Brassell 1978). A sudden onset of seemingly vague symptoms may be very frightening, so listening to patient worries, educating and counselling, while also assessing for signs of anxiety or depression, may be very important (Brown et al. 2014). Nurses should also be mindful of some the hidden effects of taking GCs, such as loss of sleep, as well as the more visible GC side effects, that is, the cushingoid 'moon' face (Cushing's syndrome), striae of arms/legs/torso and the kyphotic 'buffalo hump' that may accompany secondary spinal osteoporosis, all of which can cause additional distress for the patient with PMR, as can GC-associated weight gain with resultant reduced activity and diminishing fitness levels.

4.11.2 Symptom Management

It is unusual to need additional medication to manage PMR symptoms. While not evidence based, some patients also anecdotally report using heat therapy (hot packs, warm showers or baths) to reduce shoulder and hip aches. Additionally, promoting positive 'keep moving' messages should not only reduce PMR-related stiffness but can help prevent long-standing weakness and deconditioning quickly developed in less active older populations.

4.11.3 Medication Education

Patient priorities in PMR have been reported in a national survey (Muller et al. 2018). The highest priority for supporting people with PMR was reported to be 'being on and tapering steroids' with information being requested on the duration and benefits of steroids as well as knowing and mitigating side effects. The nurse can, therefore, play a vital educational role with these patients and can unobtrusively monitor cumulative doses, associated with higher incidence of adverse events.

Sharing with patients the known side effects of GCs and what to observe for will be an important component of early consultations for all nurses following diagnosis (Dixon and Bansback 2012). Equally important is to ensure patients understand the negative consequences of suddenly stopping the GCs, such as extreme fatigue, dizziness and light-headedness. Given PMR affects an older population with frequent polypharmacy challenges, there may also be other possible drug interactions about which the patient may need information. Onward referral to pharmacists or back to physicians for additional insights may be important.

Concerns about OP may cause the nurse to consider additional requirement for bone protection agents such as bisphosphonates, which may be given prophylactically or following a confirmed osteopaenic or OP diagnosis following a DXA scan. In PMR, these are often prescribed with a calcium and vitamin D supplement (Hennell et al. 2007), so an explanation regarding the value for additional medication will be important to optimise patient concordance.

4.11.4 Patient Education

Teaching patients to cope with PMR has been an identified nursing focus for some time (Brassell 1978). A key aspect of this will be empowering patients to be knowledgeable and confident enough to self-manage their condition. Identifying the bespoke needs of the patient will, therefore, be an important nursing role. In addition to the GC advice, other patient education will usually include the following:

(a) What is PMR; an explanation of the condition
(b) Explanation of the blood test results

(c) Minimising the impact of GC side effects; encouraging mobility, promoting weight-bearing activity
(d) Monitoring skin condition, avoiding pressure or damage
(e) How to identify relapse in PMR; symptoms to note
(f) The risk of GCA; to pay attention to visual disturbances
(g) Recognising the signs of OP
(h) Health professional follow-up contact details; helpline numbers
(i) Available patient support groups/online fora, for example, The PMRGCAuk charity (http://www.pmrgca.co.uk/content/home-page)

If available, offering ongoing support via a nurse-led telephone advice line can be very reassuring to patients, also serving to help triage and prioritise patients needing onward escalated medical management. Nurses can also signpost patients to other online and telephone support. For example, in the United Kingdom, the PMRGCAuk charity serves as a patient forum holding regular national and regional support group meetings, as well as raising increased awareness about both PMR and GCA conditions and promoting related research.

4.11.5 Multi-disciplinary Team Referrals

Referral to other health professional colleagues such as physiotherapy and occupational therapy can offer the patient further education and self-management strategies (Hennell et al. 2007) and promote maintenance or regaining of independence, all important to avoid loss of roles and keeping morale high.

Therapy referrals are likely to be most appropriate for patients who are less mobile, possibly due to other comorbidities, the ageing process, or for those struggling to achieve their usual daily activities, family or work commitments. Consideration of an individualised exercise programme to maintain strength, reduce the risk of falls and generally improve daily living may be especially relevant for patients with more established PMR (Dejaco et al. 2015; Whitlock and Hollywood 2014). Older people may experience difficulties with balance due to loss of muscle strength and joint flexibility as well as reduced vision and reaction time. Managing PMR-associated fatigue may also be helped by therapists' interventions, especially activity modification and pacing education and advice.

4.12 Prognosis and Relapse

While for many, the overall prognosis for PMR is generally very good and does not appear to affect mortality (Salvarani et al. 1995); relapsing symptoms are remarkably common and thought to affect as many as 50% of patients (Kremers et al. 2005a; Salvarani et al. 2005).

Relapse has been defined by consensus as a 'flare up of symptoms' illustrated by the patient reporting shoulder and/or hip pain (>20 mm on visual analogue scale) with a perception of shoulder pain exacerbated by activity and reduced elevation range of movement, together with an accompanying morning stiffness of more than 30 min. These indicators will often, although not always, be accompanied by abnormal CRP and ESR inflammatory markers. To minimise delay identifying possible relapse, the nurse may offer patients with PMR an urgent blood form to keep in reserve, which facilitates prompt detection of rising ESR and CRP.

Women, who start on higher GC dosages or those who taper too fast, are most likely to relapse (Kremers et al. 2005b), but actual prediction of who will relapse remains difficult. When suspecting relapse, the nurse should always first consider other causes; for example, a raised ESR associated with infection, before managing likely PMR relapse with an increasing GC dosage (Dejaco et al. 2011).

Summary of Main Points for Learning
- PMR presents as sudden onset of bilateral shoulder and hip girdle ache with stiffness and fatigue in an older person.
- 20% of people with PMR also develop GCA, which if left untreated can lead to permanent blindness.
- Glucocorticoid therapy is largely successful in achieving remission of symptoms, but has multiple side effects.
- The nurse has an important role psychologically supporting the newly diagnosed, as well as explaining and educating patients about GC therapy, including recognition of side effects.
- 50% of patients relapse while tapering GC therapy, so ongoing vigilance is needed.

4.13   Self-Assessment

Consider the following questions; reflect on what you have learnt in this chapter and how this might be relevant to your clinical practice.

1. Can you summarise the common clinical features observed in patients with PMR?
2. What questions might you ask a patient with known PMR to exclude the likelihood of GCA?
3. Identify six common side effects of taking glucocorticoid medication. Discuss with your colleagues how you currently monitor your patients for these; could this system be improved?
4. Think about the current psychological support offered to patients with PMR in your service. Thinking holistically, incorporating what PMRGCAuk can also provide, consider how you might want to alter this to enhance your patients' experience?

References

Alvarez-Rodríguez L, Lopez-Hoyos M, Mata C, Marin MJ, Calvo-Alen J, Blanco R, et al. Circulating cytokines in active polymyalgia rheumatica. Ann Rheum Dis. 2010;69(1):263–9.

Barber HS. Myalgic syndrome with constitutional effects; polymyalgia rheumatica. Ann Rheum Dis. 1957;16(2):230–7.

Brassell MP. Teaching patients to cope with polymyalgia rheumatica. Nursing. 1978;8(5):22–4.

Brown S, Bond D, Waldron N. Less common rheumatological diseases: an introduction. Pract Nurse. 2014;44(9):40–6.

Bruce W. Senile rheumatic gout. Br Med J. 1888;2(1450):811–3.

Crowson CS, Matteson EL. Contemporary prevalence estimates for giant cell arteritis and polymyalgia rheumatica, 2015. Semin Arthritis Rheum. 2017;47:253–6.

Crowson CS, Matteson EL, Myasoedova E, Michet CJ, Ernste FC, Warrington KJ, et al. The lifetime risk of adult-onset rheumatoid arthritis and other inflammatory autoimmune rheumatic diseases. Arthritis Rheum. 2011;63(3):633–9.

Dasgupta B. Polymyalgia rheumatica. In: Watts RA, Conaghan PG, Denton C, Foster H, Isaacs J, Muller-Ladner U, editors. Oxford textbook of rheumatology. 4th ed. Oxford, UK: Oxford University Press; 2013. p. 1125–31.

Dasgupta B, Borg FA, Hassan N, Barraclough K, Bourke B, Fulcher J, et al. BSR and BHPR guidelines for the management of polymyalgia rheumatica. Rheumatology. 2010;49(1):186–90, 5p.

Dasgupta B, Cimmino MA, Kremers HM, Schmidt WA, et al. 2012 Provisional classification criteria for polymyalgia rheumatica: a European League Against Rheumatism/American College of Rheumatology collaborative initiative. Ann Rheum Dis. 2012a;71(4):484–92.

Dasgupta B, Cimmino MA, Kremers HM, Schmidt WA, et al. 2012 Provisional classification criteria for polymyalgia rheumatica: a European League Against Rheumatism/American College of Rheumatology collaborative initiative. Arthritis Rheum. 2012b;64(4):943–54.

De Bandt M. Current diagnosis and treatment of polymyalgia rheumatica. Joint Bone Spine. 2014;81(3):203–8, 6p.

Dejaco C, Duftner C, Cimmino MA, Dasgupta B, Salvarani C, Crowson CS, et al. Definition of remission and relapse in polymyalgia rheumatica: data from a literature search compared with a Delphi-based expert consensus. Ann Rheum Dis. 2011;70(3):447–53.

Dejaco C, Singh YP, Perel P, Hutchings A, Camellino D, Mackie S, et al. 2015 Recommendations for the management of polymyalgia rheumatica: a European League Against Rheumatism/American College of Rheumatology collaborative initiative. Ann Rheum Dis. 2015;74(10):1799–807.

Dixon WG, Bansback N. Understanding the side effects of glucocorticoid therapy: shining a light on a drug everyone thinks they know. Ann Rheum Dis. 2012;71(11):1761–4.

Duarte C, Ferreira RJO, Mackie SL, Kirwan JR, Pereira dS. Outcome measures in polymyalgia rheumatica. A systematic review. J Rheumatol. 2015;42(12):2503–11.

Falsetti P, Acciai C, Volpe A, Lenzi L. Ultrasonography in early assessment of elderly patients with polymyalgic symptoms: a role in predicting diagnostic outcome? Scand J Rheumatol. 2011;40(1):57–63.

Fardet L. Glucocorticoid-induced adverse events in patients with giant cell arteritis or polymyalgia rheumatica. Rev Med Interne. 2013;34(7):438–43.

Fardet L, Fève B. Systemic glucocorticoid therapy: a review of its metabolic and cardiovascular adverse events. Drugs. 2014;74(15):1731–45, 15p.

Frediani B, Falsetti P, Storri L, Bisogno S, Baldi F, Campanella V, et al. Evidence for synovitis in active polymyalgia rheumatica: sonographic study in a large series of patients. J Rheumatol. 2002;29(1):123–30.

Fries JF, Spitz P, Kraines RG, Holman HR. Measurement of patient outcome in arthritis. Arthritis Rheum. 1980;23(2):137–45.

Gonzalez-Gay M, Vazquez-Rodriguez T, Lopez-Diaz M, Miranda-Filloy J, Gonzalez-Juanatey C, Martin J, et al. Epidemiology of giant cell arteritis and polymyalgia rheumatica. Arthritis Rheum. 2009;61(10):1454–61.

Gran JT, Myklebust G. The incidence of polymyalgia rheumatica and temporal arteritis in the county of Aust Agder, south Norway: a prospective study 1987–94. J Rheumatol. 1997;24(9):1739–43.

Green DJ, Muller S, Mallen CD, Hider SL. Fatigue as a precursor to polymyalgia rheumatica: an explorative retrospective cohort study. Scand J Rheumatol. 2015;44(3):219–23, 5p.

Hayward RA, Rathod T, Muller S, Hider SL, Roddy E, Mallen CD. Association of polymyalgia rheumatica with socioeconomic status in primary care: a cross-sectional observational study. Arthritis Care Res (Hoboken). 2014;66(6):956–60.

Helliwell T, Hider SL, Mallen CD. Polymyalgia rheumatica: diagnosis, prescribing, and monitoring in general practice. Br J Gen Pract. 2013;63(610):e361–6.

Helliwell T, Brouwer E, Pease CT, Hughes R, Hill CL, Neill LM, et al. Development of a provisional core domain set for polymyalgia rheumatica: report from the OMERACT 12 Polymyalgia Rheumatica Working Group. J Rheumatol. 2016;43(1):182–6.

Hennell SL. Nurse prescribing in rheumatology: a case study. Musculoskeletal Care. 2004;2(1):65–71.

Hennell S, Busteed S, George E. Evidence-based management for polymyalgia rheumatica for rheumatology practitioners, nurses and physiotherapists. Musculoskeletal Care. 2007;5(2):65–71.

Kennedy-Malone L, Enevold GL. Assessment and management of polymyalgia rheumatica in older adults. Geriatr Nurs. 2001;22(3):152–5.

Kermani TA, Warrington KJ. Polymyalgia rheumatica. Lancet. 2013;381(9860):63–72. North American Edition, 10p.

Kreiner F, Langberg H, Galbo H. Increased muscle interstitial levels of inflammatory cytokines in polymyalgia rheumatica. Arthritis Rheum. 2010;62(12):3768–75.

Kremers HM, Reinalda MS, Crowson CS, Zinsmeister AR, Hunder GG, Gabriel SE. Relapse in a population based cohort of patients with polymyalgia rheumatica. J Rheumatol. 2005a;32(1):65–73.

Kremers HM, Reinalda MS, Crowson CS, Zinsmeister AR, Hunder GG, Gabriel SE. Use of physician services in a population-based cohort of patients with polymyalgia rheumatica over the course of their disease. Arthritis Rheum. 2005b;53(3):395–403.

Leslie M, Fitzgerald DC, Mikanowicz C. Musculoskeletal aching in the older adult: polymyalgia rheumatica and giant cell arteritis. Top Adv Pract Nurs. 2003;3(1):5p.

Macchioni P, Boiardi L, Catanoso M, Pazzola G, Salvarani C. Performance of the new 2012 EULAR/ACR classification criteria for polymyalgia rheumatica: comparison with the previous criteria in a single-centre study. Ann Rheum Dis. 2014;73(6):1190–3.

Mackie SL, Mallen CD. Polymyalgia rheumatica. BMJ. 2013;347:f6937.

Mackie SL, Pease CT. Diagnosis and management of giant cell arteritis and polymyalgia rheumatica: challenges, controversies and practical tips. Postgrad Med J. 2013;89(1051):284–92.

Mackie SL, Arat S, da Silva J, Duarte C, Halliday S, Hughes R, et al. Polymyalgia Rheumatica (PMR) Special Interest Group at OMERACT 11: outcomes of importance for patients with PMR. J Rheumatol. 2014;41(4):819–23.

Muller S, Hider SL, Belcher J, Helliwell T, Mallen CD. Is cancer associated with polymyalgia rheumatica? A cohort study in the General Practice Research Database. Ann Rheum Dis. 2014;73(10):1769–73.

Muller S, Hider SL, Helliwell T, Lawton S, Barraclough K, Dasgupta B, et al. Characterising those with incident polymyalgia rheumatica in primary care: results from the PMR Cohort Study. Arthritis Res Ther. 2016;18:200.

Muller S, O'Brien A, Helliwell T, Hay CA, Gilbert K, Mallen CD, et al. Support available for and perceived priorities of people with polymyalgia rheumatica and giant cell arteritis: results of the PMRGCAuk members' survey 2017. Clin Rheumatol. 2018;37(12):3411–8.

Owen CE, Buchanan RRC, Hoi A. Recent advances in polymyalgia rheumatica. Intern Med J. 2015;45(11):1102–8.

Partington R, Helliwell T, Muller S, Abdul Sultan A, Mallen C. Comorbidities in polymyalgia rheumatica: a systematic review. Arthritis Res Ther. 2018a;20(1):258.

Partington RJ, Muller S, Helliwell T, Mallen CD, Sultan AA, Abdul Sultan A. Incidence, prevalence and treatment burden of polymyalgia rheumatica in the UK over two decades: a population-based study. Ann Rheum Dis. 2018b;77(12):1750–6.

Paskins Z, Whittle R, Sultan AA, Muller S, Blagojevic-Bucknall M, Helliwell T, et al. Risk of fracture among patients with polymyalgia rheumatica and giant cell arteritis: a population-based study. BMC Med. 2018;16(1):4.

Petri H, Nevitt A, Sarsour K, Napalkov P, Collinson N. Incidence of giant cell arteritis and characteristics of patients: data-driven analysis of comorbidities. Arthritis Care Res (Hoboken). 2015;67(3):390–5.

Raheel S, Shbeeb I, Crowson CS, Matteson EL. Epidemiology of polymyalgia rheumatica 2000–2014 and examination of incidence and survival trends over 45 years: a population-based study. Arthritis Care Res (Hoboken). 2017;69(8):1282–5.

Ruta S, Rosa J, Navarta DA, Saucedo C, Catoggio LJ, Monaco RG, et al. Ultrasound assessment of new onset bilateral painful shoulder in patients with polymyalgia rheumatica and rheumatoid arthritis. Clin Rheumatol. 2012;31(9):1383–7.

Sakellariou G, Iagnocco A, Riente L, Ceccarelli F, Carli L, Di Geso L, et al. Ultrasound imaging for the rheumatologist XLIII. Ultrasonographic evaluation of shoulders and hips in patients with polymyalgia rheumatica: a systematic literature review. Clin Exp Rheumatol. 2013;31(1):1–7.

Salvarani C, Macchioni PL, Tartoni PL, Rossi F, Baricchi R, Castri C, et al. Polymyalgia rheumatica and giant cell arteritis: a 5-year epidemiologic and clinical study in Reggio Emilia, Italy. Clin Exp Rheumatol. 1987;5(3):205–15.

Salvarani C, Gabriel SE, O'Fallon WM, Hunder GG. Epidemiology of polymyalgia rheumatica in Olmsted County, Minnesota, 1970–1991. Arthritis Rheum. 1995;38(3):369–73.

Salvarani C, Cantini F, Niccoli L, Macchioni P, Consonni D, Bajocchi G, et al. Acute-phase reactants and the risk of relapse/recurrence in polymyalgia rheumatica: a prospective follow up study. Arthritis Rheum. 2005;53(1):33–8.

Salvarani C, Cantini F, Hunder GG. Polymyalgia rheumatica and giant-cell arteritis. Lancet. 2008;372(9634):234–45.

Salvarani C, Barozzi L, Boiardi L, Pipitone N, Bajocchi GL, Macchioni PL, et al. Lumbar interspinous bursitis in active polymyalgia rheumatica. Clin Exp Rheumatol. 2013;31(4):526–31.

Seitz M. Polymyalgia rheumatica: what is the current status? Z Rheumatol. 2015;74(6):507–10.

Shbeeb I, Challah D, Raheel S, Crowson CS, Matteson EL. Comparable rates of glucocorticoid associated adverse events in patients with polymyalgia rheumatica and comorbidities in the general population. Arthritis Care Res (Hoboken). 2018;70(4):643–7.

Smeeth L, Cook C, Hall AJ. Incidence of diagnosed polymyalgia rheumatica and temporal arteritis in the United Kingdom, 1990–2001. Ann Rheum Dis. 2006;65(8):1093–8.

Straub RH, Cutolo M. Further evidence for insufficient hypothalamic-pituitary-glandular axes in polymyalgia rheumatica. J Rheumatol. 2006;33(7):1219–23.

Twohig H, Mitchell C, Mallen C, Adebajo A, Mathers N. 'I suddenly felt I'd aged': a qualitative study of patient experiences of polymyalgia rheumatica (PMR). Patient Educ Couns. 2015;98(5):645–50.

Van Staa TP, Laan RF, Barton IP, Cohen S, Reid DM, Cooper C. Bone density threshold and other predictors of vertebral fracture in patients receiving oral glucocorticoid therapy. Arthritis Rheum. 2003;48(11):3224–9.

Vivekanantham A, Blagojevic-Bucknall M, Clarkson K, Belcher J, Mallen CD, Hider SL. How common is depression in patients with polymyalgia rheumatica? Clin Rheumatol. 2018;37(6):1633–8.

Whitlock M, Hollywood J. Treatment guidelines for polymyalgia rheumatica: the nursing perspective. Rheumatology. 2014;53:i10.

Yates M, Graham K, Watts RA, MacGregor AJ. The prevalence of giant cell arteritis and polymyalgia rheumatica in a UK primary care population. BMC Musculoskelet Disord. 2016;17:285.

Further Reading

American College of Rheumatology: PMR homepage. Available from: https://www.rheumatology.org/I-Am-A/Patient-Caregiver/Diseases-Conditions/Polymyalgia-Rheumatica. Accessed 02 Apr 19.

Arthritis Foundation. Available from: http://www.arthritis.org/.

Dasgupta B, Raine C. Polymyalgia rheumatica, Section 18, Chapter 134: Polymyalgia rheumatica. In: Watts RA, Conaghan PG, Denton C, Foster H, Isaacs J, Müller-Ladner U, editors. Oxford textbook of rheumatology. 4th ed. Oxford: Oxford University Press; 2018. https://doi.org/10.1093/med/9780199642489.003.0134_update_001. Accessed 02 Apr 19.

PMR and GCA patient peer support. Available from: https://healthunlocked.com/pmrgcauk. Accessed 02 Apr 19.

PMRGCAuk Patient support charity homepage. Available from: http://www.pmrgca.co.uk/content/home-page. Accessed 02 Apr 19.

Support groups for patients in Europe. Available from: https://www.eular.org/pare_member_orgs.cfm.

Versus Arthritis: Patient information about PMR. Available from: https://www.versusarthritis.org/about-arthritis/conditions/polymyalgia-rheumatica-pmr/?gclid=EAIaIQobChMI0OLlmK2v4QIVSZPtCh3TtgSREAAYASAAEgL_-_D_BwE. Accessed 02 Apr 19.

Versus Arthritis: Steroid tablets information booklet. Available from: https://www.versusarthritis.org/media/1362/steroid-tablets-information-booklet.pdf. Accessed 10 Apr 19.

Versus Arthritis: Steroid drug treatment information. Available from: https://www.versusarthritis.org/about-arthritis/treatments/drugs/steroids/. Accessed 10 Apr 19.

Osteoporosis and Fractures

Andréa Ascenção Marques

5.1 Learning Outcomes

Having read this chapter, the reader will be able to:

1. Explain what osteoporosis is and how it is diagnosed
2. Identify the cause and risk factors for osteoporosis and fractures
3. Describe the management of osteoporosis
4. Identify how to prevent falls and reduce the risk of fractures in older people

5.2 Introduction to Osteoporosis and Osteoporotic Fracture

Osteoporosis is a condition that weakens bones, making them fragile and more likely to fracture (Fig. 5.1). Osteoporosis develops slowly over several years and is often only diagnosed when a minor fall or sudden impact causes a bone fracture (Schousboe et al. 2013).

For epidemiological purposes, fractures are designated as osteoporotic when they occur after the age of 50 years and result from mechanical forces that would not normally result in a fracture (low-level trauma) (Schousboe et al. 2013; Kanis et al. 2001). Osteoporotic fractures can also be described as "fragility fractures." Trauma is considered "low level" when its intensity is equivalent to that of a fall from standing height or less (Melton et al. 1997). An osteoporotic or fragility fracture does not occur as a consequence of other pathological causes, such as bone metastasis or primary tumors (Melton et al. 1997).

A. A. Marques (✉)
Rheumatology Department, Centro Hospitalar e Universitário de Coimbra, Nursing School of Coimbra, Coimbra, Portugal

© Springer Nature Switzerland AG 2020
S. Ryan (ed.), *Nursing Older People with Arthritis and other Rheumatological Conditions*, Perspectives in Nursing Management and Care for Older Adults, https://doi.org/10.1007/978-3-030-18012-6_5

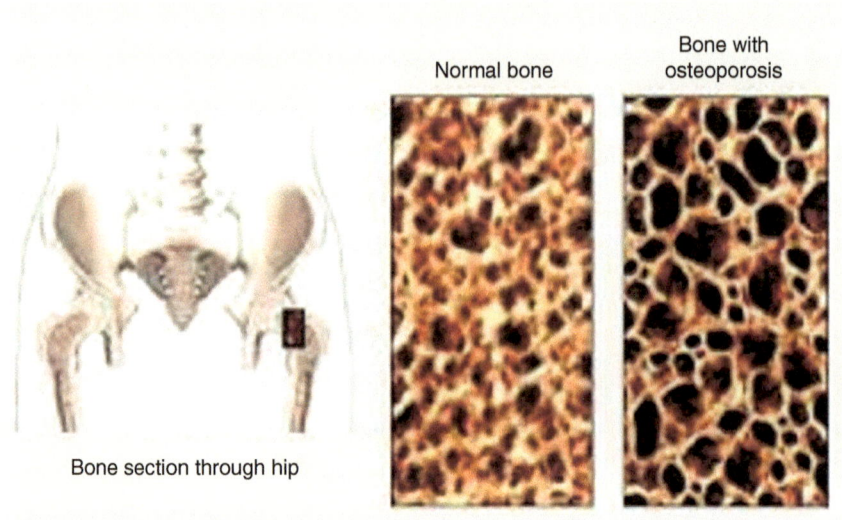

Fig. 5.1 The difference between normal bone and bone with osteoporosis

The vast majority of hip, forearm, vertebral or humeral fractures occurring after 50 years of age are due to low impact injuries and are generally considered to be osteoporotic fractures (Mackey et al. 2007). Fractures occurring in other sites, including the ribs, tibia, and pelvis, are more difficult to define as osteoporotic (Sambrook and Cooper 2006).

5.3 Cause

Bone is a biologically active tissue that undergoes continuous renovation, with osteoblasts involved in bone formation and osteoclasts reabsorbing bone. Bone matrix is essentially composed of type I collagen and calcium salts, mainly hydroxy-apatite (Schousboe et al. 2013).

During the first decades of life, bones increase in size and in mineral content, with bone mineral density (BMD) reaching a peak between 20 and 30 years of age. In the absence of other conditions, BMD remains relatively stable until the menopause in women and around 50 years of age in men. From then onward, due to the lack of estrogens and other factors related to aging, bone resorption occurs more often than bone formation. BMD decreases progressively, resulting in bone becoming more fragile. This can lead to a bone fracture following a low-intensity trauma. In females, this process is accelerated by a period of rapid bone loss that occurs after the menopause. Peak bone mass, which dependent on genetics and a healthy lifestyle in childhood and adolescence, is a major determinant of BMD later in life (Silva 2005). The difference in bone mineral density between genders is shown in Fig. 5.2.

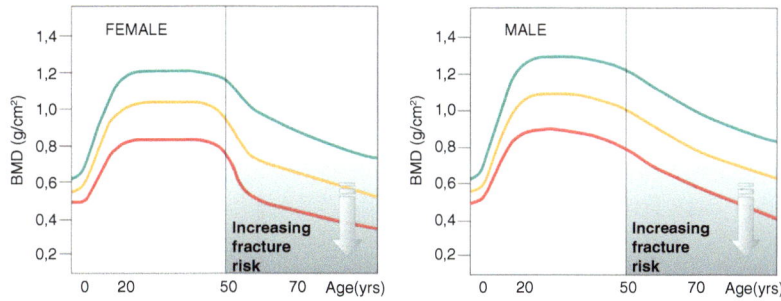

Fig. 5.2 Change in bone mass for women and men during lifetime. (Reproduced from Silva (2005))

Table 5.1 WHO criteria for diagnosis of osteoporosis

BMD T-score	Diagnosis
≥−1	Normal
−1 to −2.5	Low bone mass
≤−2.5	Osteoporosis
≤−2.5 with existing fracture	Severe osteoporosis

5.4 Diagnosis

In 1992, the World Health Organization (WHO), having recognized osteoporosis as an established and well-defined disease, established a consensus group to evaluate methods for fracture risk assessment and their suitability for use in screening of osteoporosis. As a result, diagnostic criteria for osteoporosis were published in 1994, based on the measurement of bone mineral density (BMD), which is still generally accepted. This definition is based on BMD, recognizing the strong inverse relationship between bone mineral density and fracture risk (NIH Consensus Development Panel on Osteoporosis Prevention, Diagnosis, and Therapy 2001).

A BMD T-score ≤ −2.5, measured by dual-energy X-ray absorptiometry (DXA), was the cut-off point used to define osteoporosis. The WHO criteria for different definitions relevant to osteoporosis are shown in Table 5.1.

However, this is an operational diagnosis: several other conditions, other than osteoporosis, may reduce BMD, such as osteomalacia, tumor infiltration (e.g., multiple myeloma), or renal osteodystrophy.

5.5 Signs and Symptoms

There are often no symptoms in the early stages of bone loss (Johnell et al. 2005). But once bones have been effected by osteoporosis, signs and symptoms may include the following:

- Back pain, caused by a fractured or collapsed vertebra
- Loss of height over time
- A stooped posture
- A bone fracture that occurs much more easily than expected

5.6　Risk Factors

The main risk factors for osteoporosis and osteoporotic fractures are described in Table 5.2 (NIH Consensus Development Panel on Osteoporosis Prevention, Diagnosis, and Therapy 2001).

Low bone mineral density. Low BMD (measured with DXA) is one of the most important risk factors for fragility fractures (Marshall et al. 1996). It is considered to be both nonmodifiable and modifiable since it is determined by a wide range of factors, including genetics, age, gender, and lifestyle factors (Golob and Laya 2015).

Bone mineral density is also pivotal because it mediates a substantial part of the impact of the factors described below (Kanis 2002). However, the following factors have been shown to influence the risk of fracture independently of BMD (Kanis et al. 2005a, 2007b).

Age. The frequency of fractures, especially at the hip, increases exponentially with age, especially after the age of 70 years, in both men and women, in most regions of the world (Kanis et al. 2012). Forearm fractures show an increase in incidence in white women between the ages of 45 and 60 years, while the incidence of hip fractures steadily increases with age. This has been attributed to the deterioration in neuromuscular reflexes with aging; younger people tend to use their hands to break a fall, resulting in wrist fractures, while older people tend to fall sideways or backward. This incidence of vertebral fractures reduces in older adults. This may be

Table 5.2 Nonmodifiable and modifiable risk factors for osteoporotic fractures

Nonmodifiable risk factors	Modifiable risk factors
Low bone mineral density (Johnell et al. 2005; Marshall et al. 1996)	Low bone mineral density (Johnell et al. 2005; Marshall et al. 1996)
Age (Kanis et al. 2012)	Body mass index (De Laet et al. 2005)
Gender (women) (Kanis et al. 2007a, 2012)	Smoking (Kanis et al. 2005a)
Ethnicity (Caucasian) (Kanis et al. 2012; Cauley 2011; Cauley et al. 2007)	Excessive alcohol intake (Kanis et al. 2005b)
Parent hip fractures (Kanis et al. 2004a)	Sedentary lifestyle (Julian-Almarcegui et al. 2015; Kemmler et al. 2013; Carter et al. 2001)
Secondary causes of osteoporosis (Kanis et al. 2007a)	Falls (Morrison et al. 2013)
Rheumatoid arthritis (Kanis et al. 2007a; van Staa et al. 2006)	Low intake of calcium (Kanis et al. 2005c)
Chronic corticosteroid therapy (Kanis et al. 2004b; van Staa et al. 2002)	Vitamin D deficiency (Boonen et al. 2006; Reid et al. 2014)
Previous osteoporotic fractures (Kanis et al. 2004a; Klotzbuecher et al. 2000)	

explained by the fact that vertebral fractures are frequently asymptomatic, and only about one third of these patients come to medical attention and have radiographic confirmation of such fractures (Felsenberg et al. 2002).

BMD reaches a peak by the third decade of life and decreases progressively after the fifth decade until the end of life, in both men and women (Fig. 5.2) (Hippisley-Cox and Coupland 2009). The increase in fracture risk associated with age is, however, much more intense than could be explained by BMD alone. Other changes affecting the mechanical resistance of bone and the age-related increase in falls are considered responsible for this BMD-independent effect of aging (Sambrook and Cooper 2006).

Gender. Being female, especially over the age of 50 years (NIH Consensus Development Panel on Osteoporosis Prevention, Diagnosis, and Therapy 2001), is a risk factor for fracture influenced by the smaller section and cortical thickness of female bones (Melton et al. 1992). In addition, women live longer than men, on average, which adds to the proportion of around three females to one male who experience fragility fractures (Kanis et al. 2012).

Ethnicity (Caucasian). Substantial differences have been shown in fracture incidence rates across different ethnic groups (Kanis et al. 2012). In the United States, the remaining lifetime risk of hip fracture at age 50 years is 15.8% and 6.0% in Caucasian women and men, respectively, compared to 2.4% and 1.9% in Chinese women and men and 8.5% and 3.8% in Hispanic women and men (Kanis et al. 2002). Similar ethnic and race variability in women is observed for all fractures, with annualized rates greater than 2% for white and Native American women and lower rates for African American, Hispanic, and Asian women (Fig. 5.3).

Parent hip fractures. A history of a fragility hip fracture in one of the parents is associated with significantly increased risk of any osteoporotic fracture in men and women, and this is largely independent of the BMD value (Kanis et al. 2004a).

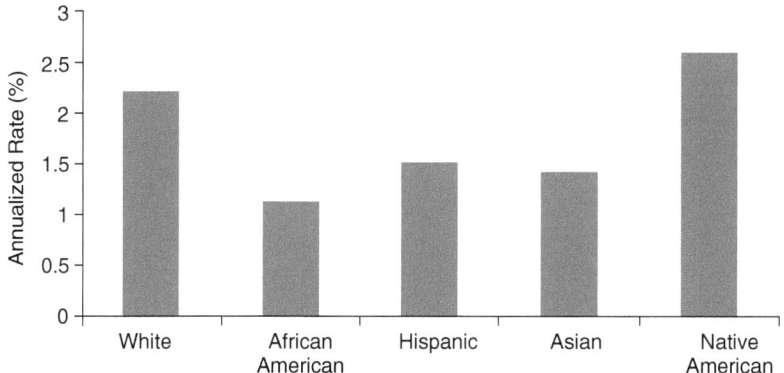

Fig. 5.3 The graph shows annualized rates of fracture by race/ethnicity according to the Women's Health Initiative Observational Study. (Derived from Cauley et al. (2007) as reproduced from Cauley (2011))

Secondary causes of osteoporosis. There are a number of clinical disorders that affect bone density and the risk of fractures (Fitzpatrick 2002). This includes type I diabetes (insulin treated), *osteogenesis imperfecta* in adults, untreated long-standing hyperthyroidism, hypogonadism, premature menopause (<45 years), chronic malnutrition, or malabsorption and chronic liver disease (Kanis et al. 2007a). The true incidence of secondary causes of osteoporosis is controversial, but several studies have estimated that it may be relevant in 20–30% of postmenopausal women and in more than 50% of men with osteoporosis (Fitzpatrick 2002; Deutschmann et al. 2002). The impact of these conditions upon the risk of fracture is partly independent from BMD.

Rheumatoid arthritis. Patients with rheumatoid arthritis have a twofold increase for osteoporosis when compared to individuals of the same age and sex who do not have RA (Kanis et al. 2007a; Cortet et al. 1995). The relative risk of fracture associated with RA has been estimated at 1.6–2.0 for hip, 2.4 for vertebral fractures, and 1.5 for fractures of the humerus (van Staa et al. 2006; Kim et al. 2010). This increased risk may be explained by several factors, including reduced exercise, lack of sun exposure, use of glucocorticoids, and the catabolic effects of circulating inflammatory mediators (Mullen and Saag 2015; Bijlsma et al. 2003).

Previous osteoporotic fractures. A history of a previous osteoporotic fracture significantly increases the risk of subsequent ones, independently of BMD (Klotzbuecher et al. 2000; Kanis et al. 2004c; Giangregorio and Leslie 2010). The risk is especially high in the months following the initial fracture and increases with the number of previous fractures. This underlines the need to establish appropriate and timely antifracture treatment in people who have experienced a fragility fracture.

Glucocorticoid therapy. Bone loss and increased rate of fractures occur early after the initiation of glucocorticoid therapy and are related to the dosage and duration of treatment (Kanis et al. 2004b), although there seems to be no safe dose in this respect (van Staa et al. 2002). The rate of fractures in steroid-treated patients is higher than expected on the basis of BMD loss alone (Goemaere et al. 2003).

Body mass index (BMI). The age-adjusted risk for any type of fracture increases significantly with lower BMI (De Laet et al. 2005).

Smoking. Smoking is associated with a significantly increased risk of fragility fractures in men and women (Kanis et al. 2005a). On the basis of observational studies, the effects of smoking on the skeleton are at least partially reversible (Hoidrup et al. 2000).

Alcohol. Alcohol consumption (≥ 3 units per day) is associated with a reduction in bone density and an increased risk of fracture (Kanis et al. 2005b; Golob and Laya 2015). These effects are mediated through direct, endocrine, metabolic, and nutritional effects that converge on the bone (Maurel et al. 2012). Evidence is scarce regarding the reversibility of fracture risk upon reduction of excessive alcohol intake (Kanis et al. 2005b).

Sedentary lifestyle. Physical activity and fitness reduce the risk of osteoporosis and fracture as well as other fall-related injuries (Julian-Almarcegui et al. 2015; Kemmler et al. 2013; Carter et al. 2001).

Falls. More than 90% of osteoporotic fractures occur following a fall (Morrison et al. 2013), and the self-reported number of falls during the previous year is associated with an increased risk of osteoporotic fractures. Every year, an estimated 30–40% of patients over the age of 65 years will fall at least once (Ambrose et al. 2015).

Vitamin D deficiency. Vitamin D deficiency is extremely common among adults and has been shown to aggravate bone loss and cause muscle weakness, thus increasing the risk of fracture (Autier et al. 2014). Vitamin D can be obtained essentially through exposure to sunlight or food supplements (Reid et al. 2014).

Low intake of calcium. Calcium is an essential component of bone. The mean daily requirement has been estimated at 20 mmol (800 mg) per day in Western diets (Ross et al. 2011). Vitamin D is essential for the absorption of calcium. A chronically low intake of calcium induces hyperparathyroidism with increased bone resorption and risk of fracture (Kanis et al. 2005c).

5.7   Investigations

Several therapeutic options and screening strategies are available (Nayak et al. 2014). The main clinical challenge remains in identifying and selecting individuals for bone densitometry and for pharmacological treatment (Consensus 2001).

Until recently, the strategy to prevent fractures was essentially based on DXA results and verification of the WHO densitometric criteria: those individuals with normal or osteopenic values were given preventive measures and individuals with osteoporosis were additionally eligible for pharmacological treatment (WHO 1994). Clinical decisions, however, must be based on absolute risks of an event, and these could only be obtained if the relative risks were applied upon the background epidemiology of fragility fractures in a similar context. This had led to the development of risk assessment tools, which can be used to estimate the future absolute fracture risk in the individual patient, based on clinical variables, with or without DXA. The most widely used of these measures is the FRAX®, but others have been developed, including the QFracture® and the Garvan risk calculator (Kanis et al. 2016).

The FRAX®, launched in 2008, was developed by the Centre for Metabolic Bone Diseases at Sheffield, in the United Kingdom (UK). It is an algorithm that estimates the probability of a fragility fracture occurring in a given individual over the subsequent 10 year, based on clinical risk factors (age, body mass index and dichotomized risk factors comprising prior fragility fracture, parental history of hip fracture, current tobacco smoking, long-term use of oral glucocorticoids, rheumatoid arthritis, causes of secondary osteoporosis, and alcohol consumption) (Kanis et al. 2007a). It may be performed with or without information on BMD and takes into account mortality in the same population, as a competing risk.

This algorithm is available online, with country-specific calibration to the national epidemiology of fracture and mortality of many countries. A systematic literature review regarding intervention thresholds based on FRAX® found that more than 120 guidelines or academic papers incorporated FRAX® for decision making in clinical practice (Kanis et al. 2016).

5.8 Management

The prevention of osteoporosis and osteoporotic fractures, both at an individual and societal levels, encompasses both nonpharmacologic and pharmacologic interventions.

Nonpharmacologic measures include the education of patients (see Chapter 12) and the general population regarding the origins of osteoporosis, with emphasis on modifiable risk factors related to lifestyle, and its consequences—fractures, death, and disability. The promotion of bone-healthy behaviors, capable of decreasing the risk of osteoporosis, falls, and fractures, is paramount in this respect (Kanis et al. 2005b).

They include adequate calcium and vitamin D intake (or sun exposure), regular weight-bearing exercise (see Chapter 10), avoiding smoking and excess alcohol intake, and, finally, measures to prevent falls (Sambrook and Cooper 2006). An important aspect, especially at the societal level of intervention, is the promotion of similar healthy habits in children and adolescents as they are essential to assure the attainment of the highest possible peak bone mass early in life (Lorentzon and Cummings 2015). All persons should be encouraged to adopt a healthy balanced diet and a physically active lifestyle beginning from childhood and continuing throughout life, in order to guarantee normal skeletal growth and aging.

Regarding pharmacologic treatment options, there are a variety of medications with different routes and dosing regimens (Table 5.3). They include bisphosphonates

Table 5.3 Pharmacological interventions used in the European Union for the prevention of osteoporotic fractures

Intervention	Year of market approval	Dosing regimen	Route of administration
Alendronate	1995	70 mg once weekly or 5 or 10 mg once daily	Oral
Etidronate	1980	400 mg daily for 2 weeks every 3 months	Oral
Ibandronate (a)	2005	150 mg once monthly	Oral
Ibandronate (b)	2005	3 mg once every 3 months	Intravenous injection
Risedronate	2000	35 mg once weekly or 5 mg once daily	Oral
Zoledronic acid	2005	5 mg once yearly	Intravenous injection
Denosumab	2010	60 mg twice yearly	Subcutaneous injection
Raloxifene	1998	60 mg once daily	Oral
Bazedoxifene[a]	2009	20 mg once daily	Oral
Strontium ranelate	2004	2 g once daily	Oral
Teriparatide	2003	20 µg once daily	Subcutaneous injection
Parathyroid hormone 1–84	2006	100 µg once daily	Subcutaneous injection

Derived from Strom et al. (2011) and reproduced from Hernlund et al. (2013)
[a]Registered but not marketed widely (Germany and Spain)

(especially alendronate, risedronate, and zoledronic acid), raloxifene, denosumab, and parathyroid hormone peptides (Strom et al. 2011). Most of these are approved only for the treatment of postmenopausal osteoporosis. However, the bisphosphonates in Table 5.3 and teriparatide are also approved for the prevention and treatment of glucocorticoid-induced osteoporosis (Lekamwasam et al. 2012) and for the treatment of osteoporosis in men (Zhou et al. 2016). Strontium ranelate was also approved for these indications, but concerns remain due to cardiovascular side effects (Soen 2016).

All these medications have been shown to reduce the risk of vertebral fracture when adequate intake of calcium and vitamin D is guaranteed. Of the available options, alendronate, risedronate, zoledronic acid, hormone replace therapy (HRT), and denosumab have been demonstrated to reduce vertebral, nonvertebral, and hip fractures.

Despite the relative efficacy of antiosteoporotic agents, systematic reviews and meta-analyses (Kothawala et al. 2007) have shown that the rate of adherence to treatment is very low: one third to one half of patients do not take their medications as recommended, with many patients stopping treatment shortly after commencing them (Kothawala et al. 2007). Nonadherence has been shown to result in an increase of risk of fracture (Imaz et al. 2010). Strategies to increase adherence, such as involving the patient in decisions about their care (Iglay et al. 2015), are required to improve efficiency.

There is consensus that the best strategy to optimize the prevention of osteoporotic fractures requires a coordinated and interdisciplinary approach. This can be enhanced by the establishment of an effective fracture liaison services (FLS). These services are usually coordinated by a dedicated nurse specialist, working in orthopedics/rheumatology under the guidance of a medical specialist in bone health. Nurses are often key to the success of these services (McLellan et al. 2003; Sale et al. 2011; Wallace et al. 2011; Ahmed et al. 2012). The implementation of such services is likely to raise awareness of osteoporosis among healthcare providers, while also undertaking patient assessment for the risk of fracture (Sale et al. 2011). Such services may also provide preventive strategies to target the general population (Akesson et al. 2013).

5.9 Managing and Preventing Falls

Falls and fall-related injuries are a common and serious problem for older people. People aged 65 years and older have the highest risk of falling, with 30% of people older than 65 years and 50% of people older than 80 years falling at least once a year (Morrison et al. 2013).

The most common cause of fractures in the older adult is falling, usually from standing height, and falling is the leading cause of hospitalization due to accidental injury, with significant risk of death in the following year due to complications (Ambrose et al. 2015).

Risk factors for falls include the following:

- Cognitive impairment
- Continence problems

- Fall history, including causes and consequences (such as injury and fear of falling)
- Footwear that is unsuitable or missing
- Health problems that may increase their risk of falling
- Medication
- Postural instability, mobility problems, and/or balance problems
- Syncope syndrome
- Visual impairment

Many measures are available to help nurses undertake screening and assessment for falls. All older people, whether living in the community or in residential care, should be regularly screened for the risk of falling. The most effective screening approach is, for it to be done routinely, if they have fallen in the past year (Ambrose et al. 2015). Several tests are available to assess the falls risk (for more detailed information, please refer to the sites indicated in the suggested further study section of this chapter).

Multifactorial intervention programs that focus of the following elements are clinically effective in reducing falls (Ambrose et al. 2015):

- Exercise/physical therapy
- Home hazard modification
- Cognitive/behavioral interventions
- Medication withdrawal/adjustment
- Nutritional/vitamin supplementation
- Hormonal and other pharmacological therapies
- Referral for correction of visual deficiency
- Cardiac pacemaker insertion for syncope-associated falls
- Exercise, visual correction, and home safety
- Multidisciplinary, multifactorial health/environmental risk factor screening and intervention (community dwelling)
- Multifactorial intervention in residential settings
- Multidisciplinary, multifactorial health/environmental risk factor screening and intervention (community dwelling)
- Multifactorial intervention in residential settings

Summary of the Main Points
- Causes and risk factors of osteoporosis and fractures
- Management of osteoporosis and fractures
- Pharmacologic and nonpharmacologic treatment of osteoporosis and fracture
- Causes of and risk factors for falling
- Role of nurses in the prevention and treatment of osteoporosis, fractures, and falls

5.10   Self-Assessment

Consider the following questions: reflect on what you have learnt in this chapter and how this might be relevant to your clinical practice:

1. Explain to a colleague how the diagnosis of osteoporosis is made
2. Identify five modifiable risk factors for osteoporotic fractures
3. Name four nonpharmacological measures used in the management of osteoporosis
4. Name four pharmacological treatments used in the management of osteoporosis
5. Explain how you would advise an older person to minimize their risk of falls

5.11   Suggested Further Study

Search for information and online programs on:

- www.nice.org.uk/guidance/CG161
- https://www.iofbonehealth.org/
- https://www.capturethefracture.org/fracture-liaison-services

Talk with patients, careers, and other staff about the interventions that can prevent osteoporosis, fractures, and falls. Reflect on what these conversations suggest about how practice might be developed to improve outcomes by involving patients.

References

Ahmed M, Durcan L, O'Beirne J, Quinlan J, Pillay I. Fracture liaison service in a non-regional orthopaedic clinic—a cost-effective service. Ir Med J. 2012;105(1):24.. 6-7

Akesson K, Marsh D, Mitchell PJ, McLellan AR, Stenmark J, Pierroz DD, et al. Capture the fracture: a best practice framework and global campaign to break the fragility fracture cycle. Osteoporos Int. 2013;24(8):2135–52.

Ambrose AF, Cruz L, Paul G. Falls and fractures: a systematic approach to screening and prevention. Maturitas. 2015;82(1):85–93.

Autier P, Boniol M, Pizot C, Mullie P. Vitamin D status and ill health: a systematic review. Lancet Diabetes Endocrinol. 2014;2(1):76–89.

Bijlsma JW, Boers M, Saag KG, Furst DE. Glucocorticoids in the treatment of early and late RA. Ann Rheum Dis. 2003;62(11):1033–7.

Boonen S, Bischoff-Ferrari HA, Cooper C, Lips P, Ljunggren O, Meunier PJ, et al. Addressing the musculoskeletal components of fracture risk with calcium and vitamin D: a review of the evidence. Calcif Tissue Int. 2006;78(5):257–70.

Carter ND, Kannus P, Khan KM. Exercise in the prevention of falls in older people: a systematic literature review examining the rationale and the evidence. Sports Med. 2001;31(6):427–38.

Cauley JA. Defining ethnic and racial differences in osteoporosis and fragility fractures. Clin Orthop Relat Res. 2011;469(7):1891–9.

Cauley JA, Wu L, Wampler NS, Barnhart JM, Allison M, Chen Z, et al. Clinical risk factors for fractures in multi-ethnic women: the Women's Health Initiative. J Bone Miner Res. 2007;22(11):1816–26.

Consensus N. Development panel on osteoporosis: prevention, diagnosis and therapy. J Am Med Assoc. 2001;285(11):785–95.

Cortet B, Flipo RM, Duquesnoy B, Delcambre B. Bone tissue in rheumatoid arthritis (1). Bone mineral density and fracture risk. Rev Rhum Engl Ed. 1995;62(3):197–204.

De Laet C, Kanis JA, Oden A, Johanson H, Johnell O, Delmas P, et al. Body mass index as a predictor of fracture risk: a meta-analysis. Osteoporos Int. 2005;16(11):1330–8.

Deutschmann HA, Weger M, Weger W, Kotanko P, Deutschmann MJ, Skrabal F. Search for occult secondary osteoporosis: impact of identified possible risk factors on bone mineral density. J Intern Med. 2002;252(5):389–97.

Felsenberg D, Silman AJ, Lunt M, Armbrecht G, Ismail AA, Finn JD, et al. Incidence of vertebral fracture in Europe: results from the European Prospective Osteoporosis Study (EPOS). J Bone Miner Res. 2002;17(4):716–24.

Fitzpatrick LA. Secondary causes of osteoporosis. Mayo Clin Proc. 2002;77(5):453–68.

Giangregorio LM, Leslie WD. Time since prior fracture is a risk modifier for 10-year osteoporotic fractures. J Bone Miner Res. 2010;25(6):1400–5.

Goemaere S, Liberman UA, Adachi JD, Hawkins F, Lane N, Saag KG, et al. Incidence of non-vertebral fractures in relation to time on treatment and bone density in glucocorticoid-treated patients: a retrospective approach. J Clin Rheumatol. 2003;9(3):170–5.

Golob AL, Laya MB. Osteoporosis: screening, prevention, and management. Med Clin North Am. 2015;99(3):587–606.

Hernlund E, Svedbom A, Ivergard M, Compston J, Cooper C, Stenmark J, et al. Osteoporosis in the European Union: medical management, epidemiology and economic burden. A report prepared in collaboration with the International Osteoporosis Foundation (IOF) and the European Federation of Pharmaceutical Industry Associations (EFPIA). Arch Osteoporos. 2013;8(1–2):136.

Hippisley-Cox J, Coupland C. Predicting risk of osteoporotic fracture in men and women in England and Wales: prospective derivation and validation of QFractureScores. BMJ. 2009;339(7733):1291–5.

Hoidrup S, Prescott E, Sorensen TI, Gottschau A, Lauritzen JB, Schroll M, et al. Tobacco smoking and risk of hip fracture in men and women. Int J Epidemiol. 2000;29(2):253–9.

Iglay K, Cao X, Mavros P, Joshi K, Yu S, Tunceli K. Systematic literature review and meta-analysis of medication adherence with once-weekly versus once-daily therapy. Clin Ther. 2015;37(8):1813–21.e1.

Imaz I, Zegarra P, Gonzalez-Enriquez J, Rubio B, Alcazar R, Amate JM. Poor bisphosphonate adherence for treatment of osteoporosis increases fracture risk: systematic review and meta-analysis. Osteoporos Int. 2010;21(11):1943–51.

Johnell O, Kanis JA, Oden A, Johansson H, De Laet C, Delmas P, et al. Predictive value of BMD for hip and other fractures. J Bone Miner Res. 2005;20(7):1185–94.

Julian-Almarcegui C, Gomez-Cabello A, Huybrechts I, Gonzalez-Aguero A, Kaufman JM, Casajus JA, et al. Combined effects of interaction between physical activity and nutrition on bone health in children and adolescents: a systematic review. Nutr Rev. 2015;73(3):127–39.

Kanis JA. Diagnosis of osteoporosis and assessment of fracture risk. Lancet. 2002;359(9321):1929–36.

Kanis JA, Oden A, Johnell O, Jonsson B, de Laet C, Dawson A. The burden of osteoporotic fractures: a method for setting intervention thresholds. Osteoporos Int. 2001;12(5):417–27.

Kanis JA, Johnell O, De Laet C, Jonsson B, Oden A, Ogelsby AK. International variations in hip fracture probabilities: implications for risk assessment. J Bone Miner Res. 2002;17(7):1237–44.

Kanis JA, Johansson H, Oden A, Johnell O, De Laet C, Eisman JA, et al. A family history of fracture and fracture risk: a meta-analysis. Bone. 2004a;35(5):1029–37.

Kanis JA, Johansson H, Oden A, Johnell O, de Laet C, Melton IL, et al. A meta-analysis of prior corticosteroid use and fracture risk. J Bone Miner Res. 2004b;19(6):893–9.

Kanis JA, Johnell O, De Laet C, Johansson H, Oden A, Delmas P, et al. A meta-analysis of previous fracture and subsequent fracture risk. Bone. 2004c;35(2):375–82.

Kanis JA, Johnell O, Oden A, Johansson H, De Laet C, Eisman JA, et al. Smoking and fracture risk: a meta-analysis. Osteoporos Int. 2005a;16(2):155–62.

Kanis JA, Johansson H, Johnell O, Oden A, De Laet C, Eisman JA, et al. Alcohol intake as a risk factor for fracture. Osteoporos Int. 2005b;16(7):737–42.

Kanis JA, Johansson H, Oden A, De Laet C, Johnell O, Eisman JA, et al. A meta-analysis of milk intake and fracture risk: low utility for case finding. Osteoporos Int. 2005c;16(7):799–804.

Kanis JA, Oden A, Johnell O, Johansson H, De Laet C, Brown J, et al. The use of clinical risk factors enhances the performance of BMD in the prediction of hip and osteoporotic fractures in men and women. Osteoporos Int. 2007a;18(8):1033–46.

Kanis JA, Stevenson M, McCloskey EV, Davis S, Lloyd-Jones M. Glucocorticoid-induced osteoporosis: a systematic review and cost-utility analysis. Health Technol Assess. 2007b;11(7):iii–v, ix–xi, 1–231.

Kanis JA, Oden A, McCloskey EV, Johansson H, Wahl DA, Cooper C. A systematic review of hip fracture incidence and probability of fracture worldwide. Osteoporos Int. 2012;23(9):2239–56.

Kanis JA, Harvey NC, Cooper C, Johansson H, Oden A, McCloskey EV. A systematic review of intervention thresholds based on FRAX: a report prepared for the National Osteoporosis Guideline Group and the International Osteoporosis Foundation. Arch Osteoporos. 2016;11(1):25.

Kemmler W, Haberle L, von Stengel S. Effects of exercise on fracture reduction in older adults: a systematic review and meta-analysis. Osteoporos Int. 2013;24(7):1937–50.

Kim SY, Schneeweiss S, Liu J, Daniel GW, Chang CL, Garneau K, et al. Risk of osteoporotic fracture in a large population-based cohort of patients with rheumatoid arthritis. Arthritis Res Ther. 2010;12(4):R154.

Klotzbuecher CM, Ross PD, Landsman PB, Abbott TA 3rd, Berger M. Patients with prior fractures have an increased risk of future fractures: a summary of the literature and statistical synthesis. J Bone Miner Res. 2000;15(4):721–39.

Kothawala P, Badamgarav E, Ryu S, Miller RM, Halbert RJ. Systematic review and meta-analysis of real-world adherence to drug therapy for osteoporosis. Mayo Clin Proc. 2007;82(12):1493–501.

Lekamwasam S, Adachi JD, Agnusdei D, Bilezikian J, Boonen S, Borgstrom F, et al. A framework for the development of guidelines for the management of glucocorticoid-induced osteoporosis. Osteoporos Int. 2012;23(9):2257–76.

Lorentzon M, Cummings SR. Osteoporosis: the evolution of a diagnosis. J Intern Med. 2015;277(6):650–61.

Mackey DC, Lui LY, Cawthon PM, Bauer DC, Nevitt MC, Cauley JA, et al. High-trauma fractures and low bone mineral density in older women and men. JAMA. 2007;298(20):2381–8.

Marshall D, Johnell O, Wedel H. Meta-analysis of how well measures of bone mineral density predict occurrence of osteoporotic fractures. BMJ. 1996;312(7041):1254–9.

Maurel DB, Boisseau N, Benhamou CL, Jaffre C. Alcohol and bone: review of dose effects and mechanisms. Osteoporos Int. 2012;23(1):1–16.

McLellan AR, Gallacher SJ, Fraser M, McQuillian C. The fracture liaison service: success of a program for the evaluation and management of patients with osteoporotic fracture. Osteoporos Int. 2003;14(12):1028–34.

Melton LJ 3rd, Chrischilles EA, Cooper C, Lane AW, Riggs BL. Perspective. How many women have osteoporosis? J Bone Miner Res. 1992;7(9):1005–10.

Melton LJ 3rd, Thamer M, Ray NF, Chan JK, Chesnut CH 3rd, Einhorn TA, et al. Fractures attributable to osteoporosis: report from the National Osteoporosis Foundation. J Bone Miner Res. 1997;12(1):16–23.

Morrison A, Fan T, Sen SS, Weisenfluh L. Epidemiology of falls and osteoporotic fractures: a systematic review. Clinicoecon Outcomes Res. 2013;5:9–18.

Mullen MB, Saag KG. Evaluating and mitigating fracture risk in established rheumatoid arthritis. Best Pract Res Clin Rheumatol. 2015;29(4–5):614–27.

Nayak S, Edwards DL, Saleh AA, Greenspan SL. Performance of risk assessment instruments for predicting osteoporotic fracture risk: a systematic review. Osteoporos Int. 2014;25(1):23–49.

NIH Consensus Development Panel on Osteoporosis Prevention, Diagnosis, and Therapy. Osteoporosis prevention, diagnosis, and therapy. JAMA. 2001;285(6):785–95.

Reid IR, Bolland MJ, Grey A. Effects of vitamin D supplements on bone mineral density: a systematic review and meta-analysis. Lancet. 2014;383(9912):146–55.

Ross AC, Taylor CL, Yaktine AL, Del Valle HB. Dietary reference intakes for calcium and vitamin D. Washington, DC: National Academies Press; 2011.

Sale JE, Beaton D, Posen J, Elliot-Gibson V, Bogoch E. Systematic review on interventions to improve osteoporosis investigation and treatment in fragility fracture patients. Osteoporos Int. 2011;22(7):2067–82.

Sambrook P, Cooper C. Osteoporosis. Lancet. 2006;367(9527):2010–8.

Schousboe JT, Shepherd JA, Bilezikian JP, Baim S. Executive summary of the 2013 International Society for Clinical Densitometry Position Development Conference on bone densitometry. J Clin Densitom. 2013;16(4):455–66.

Silva J. Reumatologia prática. Coimbra: Edições Diagnósteo; 2005.

Soen S. Drug therapy for primary osteoporosis in men. Clin Calcium. 2016;26(7):1047–52.

van Staa TP, Leufkens HG, Cooper C. The epidemiology of corticosteroid-induced osteoporosis: a meta-analysis. Osteoporos Int. 2002;13(10):777–87.

van Staa TP, Geusens P, Bijlsma JW, Leufkens HG, Cooper C. Clinical assessment of the long-term risk of fracture in patients with rheumatoid arthritis. Arthritis Rheum. 2006;54(10):3104–12.

Strom O, Borgstrom F, Kanis JA, Compston J, Cooper C, McCloskey EV, et al. Osteoporosis: burden, health care provision and opportunities in the EU: a report prepared in collaboration with the International Osteoporosis Foundation (IOF) and the European Federation of Pharmaceutical Industry Associations (EFPIA). Arch Osteoporos. 2011;6:59–155.

Wallace I, Callachand F, Elliott J, Gardiner P. An evaluation of an enhanced fracture liaison service as the optimal model for secondary prevention of osteoporosis. JRSM Short Rep. 2011;2(2):8.

WHO. Assessment of fracture risk and its application to screening for postmenopausal osteoporosis. Report of a WHO Study Group. World Health Organ Tech Rep Ser. 1994;843:1–129.

Zhou J, Wang T, Zhao X, Miller DR, Zhai S. Comparative efficacy of bisphosphonates to prevent fracture in men with osteoporosis: a systematic review with network meta-analyses. Rheumatol Ther. 2016;3(1):117–28.

Part II

Aspects of Care and Management

Managing Fatigue

6

Doriana Xhaxho

6.1 Learning Outcomes

At the end of this chapter, the nurse should be able to:

- Describe the causes of fatigue
- Identify the outcome measures used to assess fatigue
- List the investigations used for fatigue
- Describe the pharmacological and non-pharmacological management of fatigue

6.2 Introduction

Fatigue is a common and debilitating symptom associated with several chronic rheumatic diseases including rheumatoid arthritis (RA), polymyalgia rheumatica (PMR), ankylosing spondylitis (AS), osteoarthritis (OA) and fibromyalgia (FMS). Fatigue has a considerable impact on the quality of life, functional decline, as well as mortality of older adults with rheumatic diseases (Hardy and Studenski 2010). Fatigue is a subjective feeling and is perceived differently by different individuals. Fatigue is multidimensional incorporating physical, psychological and social aspects (Bianchi et al. 2014). Therefore, fatigue is influenced by individual characteristics, gender and cultural differences (Hardy and Studenski 2010).

D. Xhaxho (✉)
Rheumatology, Mater Dei Hospital, L-Imsida, Malta
e-mail: Doriana.xhaxho@gov.mt

© Springer Nature Switzerland AG 2020
S. Ryan (ed.), *Nursing Older People with Arthritis and other Rheumatological Conditions*, Perspectives in Nursing Management and Care for Older Adults,
https://doi.org/10.1007/978-3-030-18012-6_6

Table 6.1 Components of fatigue

Physical fatigue	Comprises physical qualities such as sleepiness, lack of energy, weakness and feeling exhausted more easily
Mental fatigue	Comprises cognitive and emotional qualities leading to reduced levels of concentration and motivation

6.3 Defining Fatigue

Pathological fatigue is defined as a subjective sensation of generalized tiredness not explained by activity or exertion and unresolved by rest or sleep (Piper 1993). Non-pathological fatigue occurs in about 14–25% of healthy individuals and it differs from pathological fatigue because it has a clear cause such as exercise, or fever and it resolves within three months of treating the underlying condition (Schneeberger et al. 2015). With non pathological fatigue tiredness is predictable and relieved by rest or sleep (Eilertsen et al. 2015). There is no consensus on the definition of fatigue (Jason et al. 2010). A clear definition, would facilitate the classification, measurement and management of fatigue in people with arthritis (Repping-Wuts et al. 2009).

Patients often separate fatigue into physical and mental fatigue. The components of fatigue are illustrated in Table 6.1.

6.4 Prevalence of Fatigue in Rheumatic Disease

The prevalence of fatigue amongst older adults with arthritis varies widely. This variation might be due to different definitions of fatigue, different research samples, for example, including subjects with co-morbidities that cause fatigue and different outcome measures utilized to measure fatigue (Eldahah 2010).

Forty per cent of older adults with OA reported clinically meaningful levels of fatigue (Murphy and Smith 2010). The prevalence of fatigue in RA ranges from 40% to 70% (Hewlett et al. 2011), in AS the range is 37.9% (Lopez-Medina et al. 2016)–76.7% (Turan et al. 2007), in systemic lupus erythematosus (SLE) the prevalence is 90% (Zonana-Nacach et al. 2000) and in FMS the prevalence is 82% (Overman et al. 2016).

6.5 Causes and Predictors of Fatigue

Fatigue is a complex phenomenon with a multifactorial aetiology.

6.5.1 Inflammation

As different rheumatic conditions use different outcome measures of disease activity, it is difficult to generalize the influence of disease activity on fatigue across the conditions. Cytokines are proteins released by cells. In some rheumatic diseases such as RA, there is an overproduction of these cytokines. These cytokines are similar to the ones produced during viral illnesses and may be related to fatigue.

The most powerful predictor of AS fatigue was disease activity (Missaoui and Revel 2006). This positive correlation might signify that fatigue is an integral part of the disease process in AS. Improvement of fatigue following biologic therapies suggests that inflammation and cytokines may have an important role in AS fatigue (Wu et al. 2015). Whether this is directly related to improvement of disease activity or indirectly through other unknown immunological pathways remains to be determined. In RA and systemic lupus erythematosus (SLE), the relation between disease activity and fatigue is inconsistent (Hewlett et al. 2008).

6.5.2 Pain and Function

Pain is a prominent symptom of rheumatic diseases. Self-reported pain and functional disability were positively associated with fatigue in several studies in RA, OA, SLE and AS (Nicholaus et al. 2013; Ahn and Ramsey-Goldman 2012; Stebbings and Treharne 2010). A possible explanation might be that coping with pain and functional disability is tiring and requires a greater effort to perform daily activities (Van Tubergen et al. 2002). Furthermore, pain interferes with sleep, consequently affecting fatigue (Aissaoui et al. 2012). Fatigue and pain in rheumatic diseases should be considered as two separate entities and managed independently (Stebbings et al. 2014).

6.5.3 Other Chronic/Long-Term Conditions and Medications

One should consider the presence of co-morbidities in which fatigue is also a prominent symptom. These conditions include multiple sclerosis, Parkinson's disease, malignancy, diabetes, thyroid disease, congestive heart failure, chronic obstructive pulmonary disease, hepatitis C and human immunodeficiency virus infection. Anaemia and dietary deficiencies, such as vitamin B12, vitamin D and iron, can precipitate fatigue in older adults (O'Connell and Stokes 2014). Some types of medications, such as antihistamines, antidepressants, beta-blockers, muscle relaxants and sedatives, may cause drowsiness and fatigue.

6.5.4 Mood

The burden of living with a chronic condition, the constant pain and the physical impairment can lead to low mood in older adults with rheumatic diseases. Depression is considered a predictor of fatigue in several studies in RA (Nicholaus et al. 2013; Matcham et al. 2015; Katz et al. 2016), OA (Power et al. 2008), SLE (Moldovan et al. 2013) and fibromyalgia (Gracely et al. 2012).

However, most of the studies were cross-sectional (Gunaydin et al. 2009; Brophy et al. 2013), therefore a cause–effect relationship cannot be established. Furthermore, fatigue might be a symptom of depression and not related to the rheumatic disease (Targum and Fava 2011), hence prospective studies are needed.

6.5.5   Sleep Disturbance

Sleep disturbance has a higher prevalence in the older adult (Uhlig and Provan 2018). Sleep disturbance and poor quality sleep are related to pain, fatigue and depression and an overall lower quality of life in older adults with rheumatic disease. Poor quality sleep can exacerbate pain by lowering the pain threshold. On the other hand, pain can affect the quality of sleep.

Pain severity, disease activity, functional disability, corticosteroid use, depressed mood and anxiety were positively associated with poor sleep quality in SLE (Ahn and Ramsey-Goldman 2012), RA (Wolfe et al. 2006), FMS (Nicassio et al. 2002) and OA in older adults (Murphy and Smith 2010; Power et al. 2008). Similarly, in AS, pain interfered with sleep, consequently affecting fatigue (Aissaoui et al. 2012).

6.5.6   Illness Perceptions

Patients' beliefs and perceptions of their illness were predictors of fatigue in RA and were considered important determinants of behaviour that could influence their coping ability (Schakel et al. 2017). However, further studies are needed in other rheumatic diseases.

6.5.7   Age-Related Physiological Changes

Fatigue can increase with ageing as a consequence of age-related decline of multiple physiological systems such as the muscle strength and function, cardiovascular, pulmonary and cognitive function (Avlund 2010). These changes may contribute to fatigue as more effort would be needed to perform daily activities.

6.5.8   Age

There is no clear association between age and fatigue in inflammatory rheumatic diseases (Nicholaus et al. 2013; Uhlig and Provan 2018). However, these studies did not focus on inflammatory arthritis in older adults. Many factors related to fatigue, such as depression, sleep disturbance and declining physical health, have a higher prevalence in older adults.

6.5.9   Gender

The evidence that fatigue is related to gender in rheumatic diseases is very weak. Overall, women self-report more physical symptoms than men and several studies have a majority of women participants since they are easier to recruit (Kroenke and Spitzer 1998).

6.6   Assessment of Fatigue

A thorough assessment of fatigue will help the health care professional (HCP) guide the patient to treat and self-manage fatigue. It is important to gain a good understanding of the patients' experiences of fatigue. The nurse should take a detailed history and discuss the following aspects with the patient during the consultation:

- What fatigue means to the individual
- What causes fatigue
- The onset, duration and pattern of fatigue
- The severity of fatigue
- Any exacerbating and alleviating factors
- The impact of fatigue of daily activities
- Discuss expectations and lay beliefs about treatment
- Medical history
- Social history
- Medications
- Mood
- Physical activity levels
- Lifestyle factors, e.g. diet, smoking, alcohol
- Sleep quality

The SMART model can be used in order to facilitate the assessment and management of fatigue. SMART is an acronym standing for Specific, Measurable, Achievable, Relevant and Time-Effective (Stebbings and Treharne 2010).

Specific—Nurses should assess fatigue independently from pain and disease activity. One should ask specifically if the patient is experiencing fatigue, for example: 'Are you experiencing fatigue?', 'Can you explain what fatigue means to you?' 'Can you describe your experiences of fatigue?'

Sometimes patients might not understand the word fatigue, therefore other words used by older adults to describe fatigue, such as exhausted, wornout, tired, lethargic, weary, and feeling rundown, might be used instead.

Measurable—The nurse should choose a validated tool in rheumatic disease to measure fatigue (see Section 6.6.1).

Achievable—The nurse should choose a relevant and realistic approach to manage fatigue, taking into consideration patients' preferences and beliefs (see Section 6.8). Therefore, it would be helpful to evaluate the patient's outlook for fatigue management, willingness to participate in strategies to reduce fatigue, and level of family and social support.

Relevance—Fatigue is considered important by older adults and impacts on them physically, psychologically and socially. The nurse should assess the impact of fatigue on the quality of life, for example, by asking 'How does fatigue affect your everyday activities?'

Time-Efficient—Time is one of the obstacles that the nurse needs to overcome during a patient consultation on fatigue. It would be helpful to incorporate measures that are time effective and can be incorporated in a consultation.

6.6.1 Self-Reported Outcome Measures for Fatigue

Fatigue is a subjective symptom, therefore, developing objective outcome measures to quantify fatigue is difficult (Hewlett et al. 2011). Various patient-reported outcome measures (PROMs) have been used to measure fatigue in rheumatic diseases. As older adults might experience fatigue differently from people of other age groups, these PROMs need to be validated in older adults with rheumatic diseases. One should take into consideration the purpose of screening for fatigue and the cognitive ability of the patient when choosing the appropriate outcome measure to use.

6.6.1.1 Single Item Scales
1. *Visual analogue scale*

    A visual analogue scale (VAS) is a horizontal 10 cm line anchored at each end by words that describe the intensity of fatigue experienced (see Fig. 6.1). The patient is asked to mark on the scale to indicate the level of intensity of his/her fatigue.
2. *Ordinal scales*

    This scale uses words instead of numbers to describe the intensity of fatigue experienced. The patient is asked to circle the words that best describe his/her fatigue ranging from no fatigue to severe fatigue (see Fig. 6.2).

While single item scales may be useful as a screening tool, it is recognized that fatigue is multidimensional (Bianchi et al. 2014). Fatigue varies over time, necessitating assessment of both the frequency as well as the severity of fatigue (Haywood et al. 2014). Multidimensional PROMs of fatigue are useful to provide a more comprehensive understanding of different aspects of fatigue.

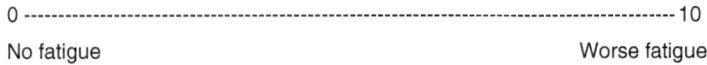

No fatigue   Worse fatigue

Fig. 6.1 A visual analogue score for fatigue

Fatigue Intensity	Score
No fatigue	0
Mild fatigue	1
Moderate fatigue	2
Severe fatigue	3

Fig. 6.2 An ordinal scale for fatigue

6.6.1.2 Multidimensional Self-Assessment Questionnaires

Numerous multidimensional scales have been used to assess fatigue in rheumatic diseases. The nurse should look at the content and practicality of the measure when choosing which PROM to use, taking into consideration the cognitive function of the older adult. Patients with fatigue might not be able to fill in a long questionnaire. The most commonly used outcome measures for fatigue in rheumatic diseases are:

- The Functional Assessment of Chronic Illness Therapy Fatigue subscale (FACIT-F) (Yellen et al. 1997)
- Multidimensional Assessment of Fatigue (MAF) (Belza 1995)
- Multidimensional Fatigue Inventory (MFI) (Smets et al. 1995)
- SF-36 vitality subscale (Ware and Shelbourne 1992)
- Fatigue Severity Scale (FSS) (Krupp et al. 1989)
- Bristol Rheumatoid Arthritis Fatigue Multidimensional Questionnaire (BRAFMDQ Bristol RA) (Nicklin et al. 2010)
- The Revised Bristol Rheumatoid Arthritis Numerical Rating Scales (BRAF-NRS V2) (Nicklin et al. 2010)

The Functional Assessment of Chronic Illness Therapy Fatigue subscale (FACIT-F) (Yellen et al. 1997) has been validated in older adults but not in older adults with rheumatic disease and measures fatigue during daily activities over the last week (Tennant 2012).

The Bristol Rheumatoid Arthritis Fatigue Multidimensional Questionnaire (Nicklin et al. 2010) assesses the overall experience, the impact and the different dimensions of fatigue. The Revised Bristol Rheumatoid Arthritis Numerical Rating Scales (Nicklin et al. 2010) measure the severity, the effect and coping with fatigue. Both outcome measures are validated in RA (Hewlett et al. 2011). Moreover, MAF (Belza 1995) and MFI (Smets et al. 1995) questionnaires are RA specific.

The Fatigue Severity Score (Krupp et al. 1989) was developed specifically for SLE patients and measures the impact of fatigue rather than the intensity of fatigue. The Fatigue Severity Score (Krupp et al. 1989) has also been used in OA, RA and FMS. There are no validated scales to measure fatigue in PMR, AS and OA.

6.7 Investigations for Fatigue

Depending on the findings of the physical assessment and history, it is essential to rule out other medical conditions that could cause fatigue. The initial screening blood tests and urinalysis might include:

- Full blood count
- Metabolic function
- Thyroid function
- Erythrocyte sedimentation rate
- Renal function tests

- Liver function tests
- Vitamin D level
- Blood glucose level
- Creatine kinase
- Ferritin, folic acid level and vitamin B12
- Screening for coeliac disease
- Urinalysis for protein, blood and glucose

6.8 Management of Fatigue

Treatment of fatigue is difficult because of its multifactorial aetiology and unclear pathogenesis. As discussed in Section 6.5.3, if there is an underlying condition that causes fatigue, it should be treated. Treatment of fatigue should be individualized and strategies used applied to all age groups (Uhlig and Provan 2018).

6.8.1 Non-pharmacological Interventions for Fatigue Management

6.8.1.1 The 4 'Ps'
The 4 'Ps' include pacing, planning, prioritizing and problem-solving and can be helpful in managing fatigue.

1. *Pacing*
   Pacing is a way to maximize one's energy while performing daily tasks. Pacing means spreading out activities, while taking frequent breaks, for example, taking a 5-min break every 30 min. The nurse might need to clarify the misconception that by pacing one performs fewer activities. In reality, pacing is helpful to perform the activities more effectively.
2. *Planning ahead*
   Encourage patients to keep a diary to plan their week and to schedule frequent breaks. The nurse can help patients to recognize fatigue patterns and adjust their daily activities accordingly. Activities that require higher levels of energy should be planned for at a part of the day when the fatigue is at a more reasonable level.
3. *Prioritizing tasks*
   It is useful to focus and prioritize activities that are important to the person. Patients can be encouraged to consider if an activity is worth doing on the day or if it can be delayed or even delegated to someone else.
4. *Problem-solving*
   Some activities can cause more fatigue than others. Patients can be supported to learn how to identify the activities that cause fatigue and alter the way these activities are performed in order to help manage the fatigue. For example, by completing household tasks such as ironing over several days.

6.8.1.2 Cognitive Interventions

Cognitive behavioural therapy (CBT) is a directive, time-limited and structured type of psychotherapy that explores the association between thoughts, emotions and behaviour (Fenn and Byrne 2013). Cognitive behavioural therapy is based on the concept that thoughts influence feelings and behaviour, hence the way of thinking can be changed in order to feel better and respond to challenging situations in a more effective way. Cognitive behavioural therapy improves self-efficacy, coping and perceptions of control. A Cochrane review (Cramp et al. 2013) showed that CBT helped to improve self-reported fatigue in adults with rheumatoid arthritis.

A randomized controlled trial (RCT) (Hewlett et al. 2011) demonstrated that RA patients who had CBT therapy showed better fatigue scores compared to controls. Age did not impact the outcomes of this study. Similarly, although CBT was not superior to usual care, a psychological intervention combining self-efficacy, social support, problem-solving and counselling reduced fatigue in SLE patients at 12 months (Greco et al. 2004; Karlson et al. 2004). There is a lack of trials on the role of CBT in the management of fatigue in other rheumatic diseases such as OA, AS and PMR. A programme combining CBT, patient education and exercise resulted in an improvement in fatigue in fibromyalgia patients (Hammond and Freeman 2006). However, most of these programmes required significant resources, hence it might be difficult to be implemented widely in clinical practice (Katz et al. 2016).

6.8.1.3 Physical Activity and Exercise

A Cochrane review concluded that physical activity, especially pool-based therapy, dynamic strength training, yoga and low-impact aerobics, improved self-reported fatigue in RA patients (Cramp et al. 2013). Similarly, graded exercise (exercise that starts very slowly and gradually increases in intensity over time) improved fatigue compared to relaxation or usual care in SLE patients (Tench et al. 2003). Another cochrane review showed that exercise improved physical function and pain of patients with fibromyalgia, but the effects of exercise on fatigue were unknown (Busch et al. 2007).

A home-based exercise programme was found to improve quality of life and reduced fatigue, in addition to medical treatment in AS patients (Yigit et al. 2013). While an intensive cardiovascular training of three sessions weekly increased fitness levels but did not reduce fatigue (Niedermann et al. 2013). However, these studies included participants of all ages and were not focused on older adults.

Feeling fatigued may reduce the motivation to exercise. Nurses should address preconceptions, beliefs and fears that the older adult may have regarding exercise.

Philips et al. (2004) suggested the following ways to motivate older adults to exercise:

- Provide education about the benefits of exercise
- Encourage manageable goals of exercising. Start exercising slowly and increase gradually
- Consider the cost/consequences of exercising (financial cost, fatigue, pain)

- Ensure that the patient feels safe during exercising (address their fears, gradual exercise progression, offer advice on joint protection and taking care of their joints)
- Consider co-morbidities that hinder exercise
- Encourage types of exercise that meet patient's demands and goals and promote socialization since several older adults may feel lonely
- Refer to a physiotherapist or occupational therapist for further guidance on exercising if required
- Taking painkillers prior to exercise
- Encourage simple exercises and day-to-day tasks such as gardening or walking to the shops

6.8.1.4 Patient Education and Self-Management Programmes

Patients need support to identify and implement changes to reduce fatigue. Patient education and self-management programmes can improve self-efficacy and lead to improvements in fatigue in RA and OA lasting up to 8 years (Barlow et al. 2009). Leaflets on fatigue and arthritis have been produced by national patient charities in the United Kingdom (see https://www.versusarthritis.org and https://www.nras.org. uk).

6.8.1.5 Sleep

As discussed in Section 6.5.5, disturbed sleep can affect pain and fatigue. Therefore, the nurse should enquire about the nature of the sleep disturbance and provide appropriate interventions to improve sleep quality. Sleep hygiene should be encouraged. Measures to improve sleep hygiene include the following:

- Having a good pillow and mattress
- Having a regular time to go to bed
- Avoiding stimulants (coffee, tea, alcohol, TV) before sleeping
- Relaxing before sleeping (a warm bath, a dark and quiet room helps)
- Avoiding lying in or taking naps during the day, as this can upset the body's natural day/night hormonal and sleep patterns

6.8.2 Pharmacological Treatment

A systematic review (Chauffier et al. 2012) and a Cochrane review (Almeida et al. 2016) concluded that biologic drugs led to a small to moderate improvement in fatigue in patients with active RA. Age did not seem to be an effect modifier on the impact of disease-modifying antirheumatic drug (DMARD) therapy on fatigue. Similarly, another systematic review (Reygaertts et al. 2018) showed small to moderate changes in fatigue in psoriatic arthritis (PsA) patients on biologic drugs.

A systematic review (O'Malley et al. 2000) showed that antidepressants may reduce fatigue in fibromyalgia. One of the reasons might be that fatigue is one of the signs and symptoms of depression. Pregabalin, an anti-epileptic drug used in fibromyalgia, has also shown significant benefit in reducing fatigue in FMS patients.

A number of RCTs in AS patients have shown improvement of fatigue following biologic therapy with anti-TNF (tumour necrosis factor) and interleukin 17-A (IL-17A) drugs (Braun et al. 2002; Sieper et al. 2015; Deodhar et al. 2016).

However, it is unclear whether the improvement results from a direct action of the biologics on fatigue or indirectly through a reduction in inflammation, disease activity or some other mechanism. The above RCTs included a small number of participants and used non-validated scales to measure fatigue. Moreover, fatigue was a secondary outcome, and the patients who had high disease activity, long disease duration and severe co-morbidities were excluded. Therefore, the participants might not be typical of patients seen in clinical practice. Fatigue is not an indicator for starting biologic drugs.

Summary of Main Points
- Fatigue is a common and debilitating symptom of rheumatic diseases.
- Fatigue is a subjective sensation of generalized tiredness, not explained by activity or exertion and unresolved by rest or sleep. Fatigue has a physical and a mental component.
- Fatigue is multifactorial with a physical, psychological and social impact.
- A patient-centred approach is required in the assessment of fatigue.
- A multidisciplinary approach combining pharmacological treatment and non-pharmacological treatment such as exercise, cognitive behavioural therapy, patient education and self-management programmes is helpful in the management of fatigue.
- Treatment of fatigue is more successful when tailored to individual needs.

6.9   Self-Assessment

Having read the chapter and undergone further study, the following are some ideas of how to relate what you have learnt to improve your clinical practice:

- Reflect on how you currently assess fatigue in clinical practice and what can be done to improve it.
- Identify outcome measures that are relevant to your area in order to assess fatigue in older adults with arthritis.
- Discuss with your colleagues the pharmacological and non-pharmacological management of fatigue and what approaches you could use in your area.

References

Ahn GE, Ramsey-Goldman R. Fatigue in systemic lupus erythematosus. Int J Clin Rheumatol. 2012;7(2):217–27.

Aissaoui N, Rostom S, Hakkou J, Ghziouel KB, Bahiri R, Abouqal R, Hassouni NH. Fatigue in patients with ankylosing spondylitis: prevalence and relationships with disease-specific variables, psychological status and sleep disturbance. Rheumatol Int. 2012;32:2117–24.

Almeida C, Choy EH, Hewlett S, Kirwan JR, Cramp F, Chalder T, Pollock J, Christensen R. Biologic interventions for fatigue in rheumatoid arthritis. Cochrane Database Syst Rev. 2016;6(6):CD008334.

Avlund K. Fatigue in older adults: an early indicator of the aging process? Aging Clin Exp Res. 2010;22(2):100–15.

Barlow J, Turner A, Swaby L, Gilchrist M, Wright C, Doherty M. An 8-yr follow-up of arthritis self-management programme participants. Rheumatology. 2009;48(2):128–33.

Belza BL. Comparison of self-reported fatigue in rheumatoid arthritis and controls. J Rheumatol. 1995;22(4):639–43.

Bianchi WA, Elias FR, Carneiro S, Bortoluzzo AB, Bertolo MB, Ribeiro SL, Keiserman M. Assessment of fatigue in large series of 1492 Brazilian patients with spondyloarthritis. Mod Rheumatol. 2014;24(6):980–4.

Braun J, Brandt J, Listing J, Zink A, Alten R, Golder W, Gromnica-Ihle E, Kellner H, Schneider M, Sorensen H, Zeidler H, Thriene W, Sieper J. Treatment of ankylosing spondylitis with infliximab: a randomised controlled trial. Lancet. 2002;359:1187–93.

Brophy S, Davies H, Dennis MS, Cooksey R, Hussain MJ, Irvine E, Sieber S. Fatigue in ankylosing spondylitis: treatment should focus on pain management. Semin Arthritis Rheum. 2013;42:361–7.

Busch AJ, Barber KA, Overend TJ, Peloso PM, Schachter CL. Exercise for treating fibromyalgia syndrome. Cochrane Database Syst Rev. 2007;17(4):CD003786.

Chauffier K, Salliot C, Berenbaum F, Sellam J. Effect of biotherapies on fatigue in rheumatoid arthritis: a systematic review of the literature and meta-analysis. Rheumatology. 2012;51(1):60–8.

Cramp F, Hewlett S, Almeida C, Kirwan JR, Choy EH, Chalder T, Pollock J, Christensen R. Non-pharmacological interventions for fatigue in rheumatoid arthritis. Cochrane Database Syst Rev. 2013;23(8):CD008322.

Deodhar AA, Dougados M, Baeten DL, Wei JC, Geusens P, Readie A, Richards HB, Martin R, Porter B. Effect of secukinumab on patient reported outcomes in patients with active ankylosing spondylitis. Arthritis Rheumatol. 2016;68(12):2901–10.

Eilertsen G, Ormstad H, Kirkevold M, Mengshoel AM, Soderberg S, Olsson M. Similarities and differences in the experience of fatigue among people living with fibromyalgia, multiple sclerosis, ankylosing spondylitis and stroke. J Clin Nurs. 2015;24:2023–34.

Eldahah BA. Fatigue and fatigability in older adults. PM R. 2010;2:406–13.

Fenn K, Byrne M. The key principles of cognitive behavioural therapy. InnovAiT. 2013;6(9):579–85.

Gracely RH, Ceko M, Bushnell MC. Fibromyalgia and depression. Pain Res Treat. 2012;2012:486590. https://doi.org/10.1155/2012/486590.

Greco CM, Rudy TE, Manzi S. Effects of a stress-reduction program on psychological function, pain, and physical function of systemic lupus erythematosus patients: a randomized controlled trial. Arthritis Rheum. 2004;51(4):625–34.

Gunaydin R, Karatepe AG, Cesmeli N, Kaya T. Fatigue in patients with ankylosing spoondylitis: relationships with disease-specific variables, depression and sleep disturbance. Clin Rheumatol. 2009;28:1045–51.

Hammond A, Freeman K. Community patient education and exercise for people with fibromyalgia: a parallel group randomized controlled trial. Clin Rehabil. 2006;20(10):835–46.

Hardy SE, Studenski SA. Qualities of fatigue and associated chronic conditions among older adults. J Pain Symptom Manag. 2010;39(6):1033–42.

Haywood KL, Packham JC, Jordan KP. Assessing fatigue in ankylosing spondylitis: the importance of frequency and severity. Rheumatology. 2014;53(3):552–6.

Hewlett S, Nicklin J, Treharne GJ. Fatigue in musculoskeletal conditions. Topical reviews: Reports on the rheumatic diseases series 6. 2008. http://eprints.uwe.ac.uk/10682/1/ARC_topic_Review_Fatigue08.pdf.

Hewlett S, Dures E, Almeida C. Measures of fatigue. Arthritis Care Res. 2011;63(S11):S263–86.

Jason LA, Evans M, Brown M, Porter N. What is fatigue? Pathological and nonpathological fatigue. PM R. 2010;2:327–31.

Karlson EW, Liang MH, Eaton H, Huang J, Fitzgerald L, Rogers MP, Daltroy LH. A randomized clinical trial of a psychoeducational intervention to improve outcomes in systemic lupus erythematosus. Arthritis Rheum. 2004;50(6):1832–41.

Katz P, Margaretten M, Trupin L, Schmajuk G, Yazdany J, Yelin E. Role of sleep disturbance, depression, obesity and physical inactivity in fatigue in rheumatoid arthritis. Arthritis Care Res. 2016;61:81–90.

Kroenke K, Spitzer R. Gender differences in the reporting of physical and somatoform symptoms. Psychosom Med. 1998;60(2):150–5.

Krupp LB, LaRocca NG, Muir-Nash J, Steinberg AD. The fatigue severity scale. Application to patients with multiple sclerosis and systemic lupus erythematosus. Arch Neurol. 1989;46:1121–3.

Lopez-Medina C, Schiotis RE, Ugalde PF, Castro-Villegas MC, Calvo-Gutierres J, Ortega-Castro R, Jimenez-Gasco R, Escudero-Contreras JC, Collantes-Estevez E. Assessment of fatigue in spondyloarthritis and its association with disease activity. J Rheumatol. 2016;43(4):751–7.

Matcham F, Ali S, Hotopf M, Chalder T. Psychological correlates of fatigue in rheumatoid arthritis: a systematic review. Clin Psychol Rev. 2015;39(1):6–29.

Missaoui B, Revel M. Fatigue in ankylosing spondylitis. Ann Phys Rehabil Med. 2006;49:389–91.

Moldovan I, Cooray D, Carr F, Katsaros E, Torralba K, Shinada S, Ishimori M, Jolly M, Wilson A, Wallace D, Weisman M, Nicassio P. Pain and depression predict self-reported fatigue/energy in lupus. Lupus. 2013;22(7):684–9.

Murphy SL, Smith DM. Ecological measurement of fatigue and fatigability in older adults with osteoarthritis. J Gerontol A Biol Sci Med Sci. 2010;65A(2):184–9.

Nicassio PM, Moxham EG, Gervitz RN. The contribution of pain, reported sleep quality and depressive symptoms to fatigue in fibromyalgia. Pain. 2002;100(3):271–9.

Nicholaus S, Bode C, Taal E, Van der Laar M. Fatigue and factors related to fatigue in rheumatoid arthritis: a systemic review. Arthritis Care Res (Hoboken). 2013;65:1128–246.

Nicklin J, Cramp F, Kirwan J, Urban M, Hewlett S. Collaboration with patients in the design of patient-reported outcome measures: capturing the experience of fatigue in rheumatoid arthritis. Arthritis Rheum. 2010;62(11):1552–8.

Niedermann K, Sidelnikov E, Muggli C, Dagfinrud H, Hermann M, Tamborrini G, Ciurea A, Bischoff-Ferrari H. Effect of cardiovascular training on fitness and perceived disease activity in people with ankylosing spondylitis. Arthritis Care Res. 2013;65(11):1844–52.

O'Connell C, Stokes E. Fatigue. In: Kauffman TL, Scott WR, Barr JO, Moran ML, editors. A comprehensive guide to geriatric rehabilitation. 3rd ed. London: Churchill Livingstone/Elsevier; 2014. p. 453–5.

O'Malley PG, Balden E, Tomkins G, Santoro J, Kroenke K, Jackson JL. Treatment of fibromyalgia with antidepressants: a meta-analysis. J Gen Intern Med. 2000;15(9):659–66.

Overman CL, Kool MB, Da Silva JAP, Geenen R. The prevalence of severe fatigue in rheumatic diseases: an international study. Clin Rheumatol. 2016;35:409–15.

Philips EM, Schneider JC, Mercer GR. Motivating elders to initiate and maintain exercise. Arch Phys Med Rehabil. 2004;85(3):S52–7.

Piper B. Pathophysiological phenomena in nursing: human responses to illness. USA: W.B. Saunders; 1993.

Power JD, Badley EM, French MR, Wall AJ, Hawker GA. Fatigue in osteoarthritis: a qualitative study. BMC Musculoskelet Disord. 2008;9:63. http://www.biomedcentral. com/1471-2474/9/63.

Repping-Wuts H, Van Riel P, Van Achterberg T. Fatigue in patients with rheumatoid arthritis: what is known and what is needed. Rheumatology. 2009;48(3):207–9.

Reygaertts T, Fautrel B, Mitrovic S, Gossec L. Effect of biologics on fatigue in psoriatic arthritis: a systematic literature review with meta-analysis. Joint Bone Spine. 2018;85(4):405–10.

Schakel W, Bode C, Van der Aa H, Hulshof C, Bosmans JE, Van Rens G, Van Nispen R. Exploring the patient perspective of fatigue in adults with visual impairment: a qualitative study. Br Med J Open. 2017;7(8):e015023. https://doi.org/10.1136/bmjopen-2016-015023.

Schneeberger EE, Marengo MF, Dal Pra F, Cocco JA, Citera G. Fatigue assessment and its impact in the quality of life of patients with ankylosing spondylitis. Clin Rheumatol. 2015;34:497–501.

Sieper J, Kivitz A, Van Tubergen A, Deodhar A, Coteur G, Woltering F, Landewe R. Impact of certolizumab pegol on patient reported outcomes in patients with axial spondyloarthritis. Arthritis Care Res. 2015;67(10):1475–80.

Smets EM, Garssen B, Bonke B, De H. The multidimensional fatigue inventory (MFI) psychometric qualities of an instrument to assess fatigue. J Psychosom Res. 1995;22:315–25.

Stebbings SM, Treharne GJ. Fatigue in rheumatic disease: an overview. Int J Clin Rheumatol. 2010;5(4):487–502.

Stebbings SM, Treharne GJ, Jenks K, Highton J. Fatigue in patients with spondyloarthritis associates with disease activity, quality of life and inflammatory bowel symptoms. Clin Rheumatol. 2014;33:1467–74.

Targum SD, Fava M. Fatigue as a residual symptom of depression. Innov Clin Neurosci. 2011;8(10):40–3.

Tench CM, McCarthy J, McCurdie I, White PD, D'Cruz DP. Fatigue in systemic lupus erythematosus: a randomized controlled trial of exercise. Rheumatology. 2003;42(9):1050–4.

Tennant KF. Assessment of fatigue in older adults: the FACIT fatigue scale (version 4). 2012. https://www.hartfordign.org.

Turan Y, Duruoz MT, Bal S, Guvenc A, Cerrahoglu L, Gurgan A. Assessment of fatigue in patients with ankylosing spondylitis. Rheumatol Int. 2007;27:847–52.

Uhlig T, Provan SA. Treating fatigue in rheumatoid arthritis: does age matter? Drugs Aging. 2018;35:871–6.

Van Tubergen A, Coenen J, Landewe R, Spoorenberg A, Chorus A, Boonen A, Van Der Linden S, Van Der Hejde D. Assessment of fatigue in patients with ankylosing spondylitis: a psychometric analysis. Arthritis Rheum. 2002;47(8):8–16.

Ware JE, Shelbourne CD. The MOS-36 item short form health survey (SF-36). Med Care. 1992;30:473–83.

Wolfe F, Michaud K, Li T. Sleep disturbance in patients with rheumatoid arthritis: evaluation by medical outcomes study and visual analogue sleep scales. J Rheumatol. 2006;33:1942–51.

Wu Q, Inman RD, Davis KD. Tumor necrosis factor inhibitor therapy in ankylosing spondylitis: differential effects on pain and fatigue and brain correlates. Pain. 2015;156(2):297–304.

Yellen SB, Cella DF, Webster K, Blendowski C, Kaplan E. Measuring fatigue and other anemia related symptoms with the functional assessment of cancer therapy measurement system. J Pain Symptom Manag. 1997;13(2):63–74.

Yigit S, Sahin Z, Eroglu Demir S, Aytan DH. Home based exercise therapy in ankylosing spondylitis: short-term prospective study in patients receiving tumor necrosis alpha inhibitors. Rheumatol Int. 2013;33:71–7.

Zonana-Nacach A, Roseman JM, McGwin G Jr, Friedman AW, Baethge BA, Reveille JD, Alarcón GS. Systemic lupus erythematosus in three ethnic groups. VI: Factors associated with fatigue within 5 years of criteria diagnosis. LUMINA Study Group. Lupus in minority populations: nature vs nurture. Lupus. 2000;9(2):101–9.

Further Reading

Sandıkçı SC, Özbalkan Z. Fatigue in rheumatic diseases. Eur J Rheumatol. 2015;2(3):109–13.
Stebbings SM, Treharne GJ. Fatigue in rheumatic disease: an overview. Int J Clin Rheumatol. 2010;5(4):487–502.

Pain Management

7

Sarah Ryan

7.1 Learning Outcomes

At the end of the chapter, the nurse will be able to:

1. Identify how pain receptors are activated
2. Compare the differences between C fibres and Alpha delta fibres
3. List the key components involved in pain assessment
4. Recognise the use of different pain measurement tools
5. Describe the role of drug therapy in pain management
6. Identify the different non-pharmacological interventions that can be used in pain management

7.2 Introduction

Pain is a predominant symptom in many rheumatological conditions including inflammatory arthritis (IA), gout and osteoarthritis (OA) (Geenan et al. 2018). Increasing age and the presence of co-morbidities increase the risk of chronic pain in older adults. The three commonest sites for pain in older people are the back, leg/knee or hips and 'other joints' (Abdilla et al. 2013). Stoicism towards pain is a common finding in this age group. There are strong associations between pain, low mood, loneliness and social isolation. Pain has been referred to as the fifth vital sign (Schofield 2018) and should be included in the assessment and management of the older person with arthritis.

S. Ryan (✉)
Midlands Partnership NHS Foundation Trust, Haywood Hospital, Stoke on Trent, UK
e-mail: sarah.ryan2@mpft.nhs.uk

© Springer Nature Switzerland AG 2020
S. Ryan (ed.), *Nursing Older People with Arthritis and other Rheumatological Conditions*, Perspectives in Nursing Management and Care for Older Adults, https://doi.org/10.1007/978-3-030-18012-6_7

Table 7.1 Components of pain

Sensory	Intensity, location and quality of pain
Affective	Emotions associated with pain
Cognitive	Thoughts associated with pain

The perception of pain is a unique experience and influenced by a multitude of different factors (Vardeh et al. 2016). Psychological factors play a key role in both the onset and progress of any pain disorder (Kumar and Elavarasi 2016). Consequently, the understanding of pain has evolved from a one-dimensional physical sensation to a multidimensional entity involving sensory, cognitive, motivational and affective qualities. Therefore, a biopsychosocial approach to pain assessment and management is required (Bevers et al. 2016).

7.3   Defining Pain

Pain has been defined as 'an unpleasant sensory and emotional experience associated with actual or potential tissue damage or described in terms of such damage' (Merskey and Bogduk 1994). The components of pain are shown in Table 7.1.

7.4   Pain Mechanisms

Pain is usually a reaction to one of the following three triggers:

- Mechanical: such as stretching of the joint capsule or alteration in normal joint structure.
- Chemical: such as the inflammatory response that can occur in the synovial (movable) joints of a person with rheumatoid arthritis.
- Thermal: the pain that is experienced when part of the body comes into contact with a hot surface resulting in a burn.

7.4.1   Pain Messages

When a pain receptor (nociceptor) has been activated, the pain message is transmitted to the dorsal horn in the spinal cord and up to the brain stem through connections between the thalamus cortex and higher levels of the brain. This activation releases chemical mediators from the damaged cells including:

- Prostaglandin
- Bradykinin
- Serotonin
- Potassium
- Substance P
- Histamine (Vardeh et al. 2016)

7.4.2 C Fibres and A Delta Fibres

The C fibres and A delta fibres transmit the pain messages in response to a noxious trigger. The fibres are present in the nociceptors and take the pain message to the dorsal horn where they terminate. From the dorsal horn, the pain message is transmitted via two main nociceptive pathways (the spinothalamic and spinoparabrachial pathways). Both fibres are associated with different qualities of pain (Vardeh et al. 2016).

A-Delta Fibres
- Have a large diameter.
- Pain messages are conducted rapidly.
- Myelinated.
- Respond to a mechanical trigger.
- Pain quality is described as sharp, localised and stinging.

C Fibres
- Have a small diameter.
- Pain messages are conducted slowly.
- Unmyelinated.
- Respond to more than one trigger.
- Pain quality is described as dull, diffuse, burning or aching.

7.4.3 Pain Gate Theory

It is well recognised that thoughts and emotions can influence how an individual perceives pain. For example if a person is low in mood or fearful about the pain becoming worse, these emotions and cognitions will often increase the intensity of the pain being experienced. To explain how thoughts and emotions increase pain, Melzack and Wall (1965) proposed that a gating mechanism exists within the dorsal horn of the spinal cord. The interplay between small nerve fibres (pain receptors) and large nerve fibres (normal receptors) within the dorsal horn determines which pain messages reach the brain (Vardeh et al. 2016). When there is more small fibre activation or only small fibre stimulation, the pain signal is sent to the brain and the individual is aware of pain. When there is more large fibre stimulation or only large fibre stimulation, then the gate is closed and the pain message does not reach the brain (Vardeh et al. 2016).

7.5 Assessment

When assessing a person's pain, there should be time within the consultation for the individual to talk about their experience of living with pain. The challenge the nurse is faced with is obtaining this information within, an often short consultation time (Schofield 2018). By giving the patient the opportunity to share their

Fig. 7.1 Observational
signs of pain in the older
person

- Facial changes: wincing and frowning
- Audible sounds: groaning
- Movements: body swaying, wringing of hands
- Emotional expressions: crying
- Interactions: withdrawal, aggressive behaviour

experience, the nurse is provided with valuable insight into how the pain started, possible contributing factors, previous treatments tried, the patient's lay beliefs and future expectations.

Key components involved in the assessment of pain in the older person with IA and OA are detailed below (British Pain Society 2007; Schofield 2018; Geenan et al. 2018):

1. Adopt a patient-centred approach and ask the patient about their pain including the impact on daily function, their ideas about the cause of their pain and their expectations and preferences for treatment. Patients can be guided and supported during the assessment by the use of open questions such as 'how would you describe the pain you are experiencing' and 'what activities are you having difficulty with due to the pain'.
2. Ask the patient directly if they are experiencing pain (making this question very clear and explicit). Older people may deny they are in pain but respond more appropriately when pain-related terms are used including 'soreness', 'aching' or 'discomfort'.
3. Observe for any indicators of pain including frowning, grimacing or rubbing hands (see Fig. 7.1).
4. Conduct a musculoskeletal examination (and if required, investigations) to understand what is causing the pain. For example, 15–20% of people with RA will have secondary fibromyalgia (Tung and Raizada 2016). If a physical examination reveals no synovitis (inflammation) but the presence of multiple tender joints, it may indicate that the pain is coming from fibromyalgia, which will require a different management approach.
5. Using a pain measure that the patient can relate to (see section on self-report measures).
6. Assess the effectiveness of any current pharmacological and non-pharmacological treatments. Also, discuss previous treatments used and the patient's beliefs about their ability to control and overcome the pain.
7. Assess current disease management for IA and OA. If IA is active, then the treatment needs to be optimised and this may require discussion with the patient's general practitioner (GP) or rheumatologist.
8. Assess pain-related physical, psychological and social factors that might be impacting on the pain (see Fig. 7.2). For example on functional ability such as walking to the shops or on social participation such as playing bowls. This can involve the use of the 4Ps (pain, performance, psychological status and past medical history) which supports a patient-centred approach to assessing pain (Wang 2014, see Fig. 7.3).

- Reduced physical fitness
- Reduced mobility
- Pain-related fear and avoidance of activities
- Beliefs and emotions regarding pain, for example, pain distress and catastrophizing
- Social factors, for example, family relationships, work, economic problems, and social role
- Sleep problems
- Presence of obesity
- Dependence on tobacco, alcohol and drugs

Fig. 7.2 Physical, psychological and social factors that might be impacting on pain

1. P=Pain: Use open questions to obtain an understanding about the nature of the pain. For example, how would you describe your pain, can you share with me a time when the pain was particularly bothersome.
2. P=Performance and function: Enquire about the impact the pain is having on the patient's life, including functional activities, mobility and self-care as well as recreational activities such as socialising with friends.
3. P=Psychological status: Find out what effect the pain is having on the patient's emotions including indications of anxiety and depression.
4. P=Past medical history. This can act as a reminder that the presence of co-morbidities could be impacting on pain, performance and psychological status and may need addressing by the general practitioner. The patient will not always be aware of what conditions are impacting on their pain. The nurse can assist here by identifying symptoms that are not directly related to arthritis, for example, neuropathic pain in patients with diabetes and signposting the patient to which services to alert to receive the appropriate input.

Fig. 7.3 Using the four 'Ps' in the assessment process

7.6 Guidelines for Pain Assessment and Management

The European League Against Rheumatism (EULAR) has developed guidelines providing principles and recommendations regarding the pain management of people with IA and OA based on findings from systematic reviews (Geenan et al. 2018). The principles of pain management are shown in Fig. 7.4.

7.7 Assessment Scales for Pain

Self-report measures are acknowledged as the most valid and reliable means to understand the experience of pain and are considered the gold standard for measuring pain in clinical practice and research (Schofield 2018).

- The assessment and treatment process should be guided by a patient-centred framework.

- The nurse should understand that any type of pain encompasses multiple and mutually interacting physical, psychological and social factors.

- The nurse should have basic knowledge of the pathology and treatment of IA and OA.

- The nurse should be able to distinguish between localised and generalised pain and should know that these two types of pain may coexist.

Fig. 7.4 The principles of pain management

There are various types of self-report measures available which can be used to measure the presence and intensity of pain on assessment as well as gauging any response to treatment (British Pain Society 2007). The type of assessment measure used will depend on the patient's cognitive ability. Outcome measures that are commonly used in people with arthritis are shown in Fig. 7.5.

7.7.1 Self-Report Outcome Measures for the Older Person

1. A visual analogue scale: This scale uses a vertical 100 mm line, with two numbers anchored at each end of the line, to denote the severity of pain. For example, 0 = no pain and 10 = worse pain possible. The patient is asked to mark on the line the intensity of their pain. This measure has high validity and reliability for older people who have no cognitive impairment (see Fig. 7.6).

- The Oswestry Disability Index (ODI; Fairbank and Pynsent 2000) and the Roland–Morris Disability Questionnaire (RMQ; Roland and Fairbank 2000) for back pain
- The Neck Pain and Disability Scale (NPAD) for neck pain (Wheeler et al. 1999)
- The WOMAC (Western Ontario and McMaster Universities Osteoarthritis Index for hip and knee pain) (Bellamy et al. 1988)
- The DASH (disabilities of the arm, shoulder and hand for the upper limb) (Hudak et al. 1996)
- The MFPDI (Manchester Foot Pain and Disability Index) (Garrow et al. 2000)

Fig. 7.5 Measures that are commonly used in arthritis management (Schofield 2018; Fairbank and Pynsent 2000; Roland and Fairbank 2000; Wheeler et al. 1999; Bellamy et al. 1988; Hudak et al. 1996; Garrow et al. 2000)

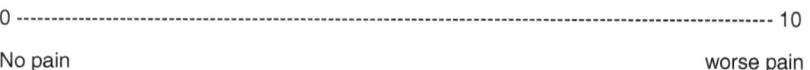

0 --- 10

No pain   worse pain

Fig. 7.6 A visual analogue score for pain

2. A verbal rating scale: This scale uses a word or a few words to describe the intensity of pain. For example, the patient may be asked to indicate the intensity of pain from the following descriptors, 'mild', 'moderate', 'fairly severe' or 'severe'. Like the visual analogue scale, this measure only provides information regarding the severity of pain and not how it makes the individual feel or the effect the pain may have on daily activities. This measure has high validity and reliability for older people who have a mild-to-moderate cognitive impairment (see Fig. 7.7).

3. A pain thermometer: Is recommended for use in older people who have a moderate-to-severe cognitive impairment, as it is easy to use. It combines the content of the visual analogue scale and the numerical verbal rating scale. It is used to measure the intensity of the pain. The validity of the pain thermometer has not been fully evaluated (see Fig. 7.8).

Pain intensity	Score
No pain	0
Mild pain	1
Moderate pain	2
Severe pain	3

Fig. 7.7 A verbal rating scale

Fig. 7.8 A pain thermometer

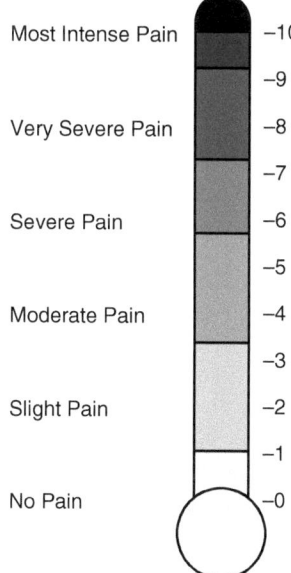

Most Intense Pain — −10

−9

Very Severe Pain — −8

−7

Severe Pain — −6

−5

Moderate Pain — −4

−3

Slight Pain — −2

−1

No Pain — −0

4. The brief pain inventory: This is a multidimensional assessment measure. It is a 15-item scale that focuses on the severity of pain, the impact on mood and enjoyment of life and the effect on physical daily activities. It has been used in older people with chronic musculoskeletal pain to identify people who are at high risk of recurrent falls (Tan et al. 2004).

7.8   Pain Management: Pharmacological

When considering advocating pharmacological treatment for the older person, it is worth remembering that sensory impairments, manual dexterity and memory difficulties all increase with age. Consequently, the nurse will need to ensure that the person can read and comprehend the drug label containing the dosage of the drug to be taken and can open the container or use a tablet blister pack, actions that can become difficult to carry out if there is a lack of power in the hands as often occurs with RA.

Physiological changes that occur with ageing can also have an effect on the action of drugs. Most drugs are broken down and excreted via the kidney or the liver. Drugs with a predominantly renal mode of excretion such as anti-epileptic drugs advocated for chronic pain need to be used with caution in patients with a compromised kidney function. The liver also becomes less efficient at drug clearance and as older people are often receiving polypharmacy drug dosages, these factors need to be taken into account when advocating medications to help with chronic pain.

A reduction in serum albumin, which is commonly seen in older people with chronic diseases such as RA and OA, affects the absorption of Non-Steroidal Anti-Inflammatory Drugs (NSAIDs) and anti-epileptic drugs increasing the potential for adverse effects to occur. Other physiological effects in the older person leading to increased fat mass, lower muscle mass and less body water can have an adverse effect on the action of medications. Homeostatic changes related to ageing can increase the risk of gastric bleeding with medications such as NSAIDs.

7.8.1   Paracetamol

Paracetamol should be considered as a first line treatment for the management of acute and persistent musculoskeletal pain due to its efficacy and good safety profile (National Institute for Health and Care Excellence 2017). A systematic review based on 13 randomised controlled trials (RCTs) concluded that Paracetamol provided short-term benefit in OA (Machando and Maher 2015). OA is characterised by periods of increased pain and when symptoms are heightened, patients should be encouraged to increase their Paracetamol dosage (within safe limits) and when the pain has settled, to reduce the dose back down to the amount that they normally take. There are few absolute contra-indications to prescribing Paracetamol. Patients should be reminded that Paracetamol can be found in many over-the-counter preparations and it is important that the maximum dose of 4 grams over a 24-h period is not exceeded. In frail older people, inadvertent overdose can be a problem with regular use.

7.8.2   Topical Treatments

Along with Paracetamol, topical NSAIDs are recommended as first line drug treatment for hand and knee OA and should be tried before oral NSAIDs are considered (National Institute for Health and Care Excellence 2017). Topical NSAIDS have a moderate effect on hand and knee pain and have the same efficacy as oral NSAIDs (Rannou et al. 2016). Consequently, NSAID gels are the treatment of choice in the older person where the risk of gastric irritation and ulceration, cardiovascular and renal side effects are increased (Rannou et al. 2016). Capsaicin is also moderately effective for OA hand and knee pain, although it can take 4 weeks before the effects are seen (Laslett and Jones 2014). Patients using Capsaicin should be advised not to take a bath after applying it or put their hands in warm water, as these actions can lead to an unpleasant burning sensation.

7.8.3   Non-Steroidal Anti-Inflammatory Drugs (NSAIDs)

Oral NSAIDs in older people should always be used with caution and only after safer treatments have been used first (National Institute for Health and Care Excellence 2017). NSAIDs are always prescribed in the lowest dose for the shortest period of time and with a proton-pump inhibitor (NICE 2014). All oral NSAIDs and cyclooxygenase-2 (CoX-2) inhibitors have similar analgesic effects but vary in their toxicity. The use of NSAIDs should be based on the taking of a full medical history and an assessment of the risk factors for the individual (National Institute for Health and Care Excellence 2017). The incidence of gastrointestinal (GI) bleeding and ulceration increases fourfold in the elderly (Sabzwari et al. 2013). Consequently, all older people on NSAIDs should be routinely monitored for gastric, cardiovascular and renal side effects. There are many drugs that are contra-indicated to use with NSAIDs including the anticoagulant Warfarin.

7.8.4   Opioids

Most prescribed opioid analgesia are given for non-cancer-related pain (Mordecai et al. 2018). The use of opioids in chronic conditions such as arthritis is not supported, especially as opioids have limited effectiveness beyond 3–4 months and are associated with the potential for numerous side effects including changes in cognition, nausea, constipation, renal failure and respiratory depression (Stannard 2013). In practice, an opioid patch may be prescribed for a short period of time if a patient was waiting for joint replacement surgery and other means of reducing pain had proved ineffective.

7.8.5 Tricyclic Antidepressants and Anti-Epileptic Drugs

Both these types of drugs have efficacy in several types of neuropathic pain but tolerability and adverse effects limit their use in older people.

7.8.6 Intra-Articular Corticosteroid Injections

Intra-articular corticosteroid injections can be effective in knee OA and reduce pain in the short term with little risk of complications. Intra-articular corticosteroid injections can provide quick and effective pain relief which can benefit function but are only effective for a few weeks to several months (Doherty and Abhishek 2018). These injections can be a useful treatment in patients who have severe arthritis changes to their joints (e.g. hips and/or knees) and have co-morbidities (such as lung or cardiac conditions) that would mean surgical replacement of the joints was not advisable.

7.9 Non-Pharmacological Interventions for Pain Management

7.9.1 Education Programmes

Patients require education on what arthritis is and the purpose of treatment, so that they have a realistic expectation as to what treatment can achieve. The emphasis should be on supported self-management and increasing the patient's confidence to try new behaviours. Education alone is not sufficient to change behaviour but it is a necessary starting point. All patients should have access to education materials and online resources (Geenan et al. 2018) (see https://www.versusarthritis.org/ and https://www.nras.org.uk).

7.9.2 Exercise

Exercises that include strengthening, flexibility, aerobic capacity endurance and balance have all been shown to be effective in older people (Abdilla et al. 2013). NICE (2014) recommends exercise as a core treatment for OA, independent of age, co-morbidity, pain severity and disability. Land-based exercise programmes have been shown to reduce pain and improve physical function in people with symptomatic knee and hip OA and can be more effective than taking Paracetamol (Iverson 2010; Uthman et al. 2013; Fransen et al. 2009). Water-based exercises can also be helpful (Iverson 2010) and by joining a local aqua aerobic class, people can also benefit from social interaction. Patient preference needs to be considered, as people are only likely to engage in exercise if they feel confident that they can do the exercise and they perceive benefit in doing exercise.

It is worth reminding the patient that there is likely to be some increased muscle ache and discomfort on starting exercise but that this will settle as their level of fitness increases. Some patients may also need to take some analgesia before they exercise to minimise the likelihood of experiencing pain.

A United Kingdom national charity (versus arthritis) produces information for patients on exercise and keeping mobile. Booklets can be obtained from https://www.versusarthritis.org.

7.9.3 Pacing and Goal Setting

Patients, who have not exercised for a while, can be fearful that any exercise will increase their pain and may cause harm to their joints. The nurse can encourage patients to start by commencing a small amount of activity initially, for example, a 10-min walk and over time as the body becomes used to this regular demand, the length of the walk can be increased or a new activity added.

Goals can be set using the SMART model (see Fig. 7.9). After goals have been agreed upon, it is important to set a time to review progress, so that goals can be modified if required and ongoing support can be provided.

7.9.4 Transcutaneous Electrical Nerve Stimulation (TENS)

A TENS machine consists of a small box with wires leading to self-adhesive pads that are placed on either side or close to the pain area. When activated, the TENS machine delivers electrical currents across the skin to block pain messages going up through the spinal cord. It can also be used to provide distraction from the pain. There is some evidence that the use of TENS can reduce pain and anxiety in older people (Abdilla et al. 2013).

S=Specific: I will go for a walk

M=Measurable: How much/how often

10 minutes 3 x a week

A=Appropriate: Something the individual wants to do

How important is the goal (1–10). If the patient scores less than 7, they need to select a goal that has a greater importance to them

R=Realistic: How confident are you that you can achieve that goal (1–10)

If the patient scores less than 7, the nurse needs to assess how their confidence level can be increased

T=Time Based: What days will you do the walk

On Monday, Wednesday and Friday

Fig. 7.9 Goal setting: using the SMART model

7.9.5   Cognitive Behavioural Therapy (CBT)

Cognitive behavioural therapy encompasses a number of behavioural and cognitive coping strategies intended to help people identify and change unhelpful patterns of behaviour and attitudes towards their arthritis (Sharpe 2016). For example, some patients can be fearful of engaging in any exercise in case it increases the pain, a concept often referred to as faulty thinking. CBT techniques can include relaxation therapy, goal setting and problem-solving to address the faulty thinking (Ehde et al. 2014). There is some evidence that CBT can reduce pain in older people living in nursing homes (Abdilla et al. 2013).

7.9.6   Orthoses

Both OA and RA can cause changes to the structure of the feet. Either by removing the fat pads under the feet so that the patient feels that they are walking on stones or glass, or in causing the toes to deviate from position, often causing friction and rubbing of the skin. Shoes should be deep and wide to prevent constricting the foot and to offer sufficient shock-absorbing properties to reduce the pressure on the knees and back. The use of flat, flexible footwear has been shown to reduce pressure, and consequently pain in the knee (Shakoor et al. 2013). If adequate footwear cannot be found, patients may need referring to an orthotist. See Chapter 11.

Some older people will have lost confidence in their walking ability and may benefit from the use of a walking aid. It is worth referring any patient who is considering using a walking aid to a physiotherapist, so that advice on appropriate aids such as a walking cane can be obtained. Purchasing the wrong aid may increase pressure on certain joints increasing the pain. Fernandes et al. (2013) found that the daily use of a walking cane reduced pain and improved function in people with OA.

Wrist splints can provide support for a joint whilst enabling the individual to remain active. If a splint is being considered, then referral to the occupational therapist will enable a full appraisal regarding the need for a splint, education on how to use it as well as advice on joint function and ergonomic principles (Geenan et al. 2018).

7.9.7   Hot and Cold Therapies

The use of hot and cold applications can be helpful in managing musculoskeletal pain. Heat is useful to reduce muscle spasm which often accompanies back and neck pain. By treating the muscle spam, this will often lead to a reduction in pain and the ability to move the affected area more easily.

Heat applications can include hotwater bottles or wheat bags warmed up in the microwave. When advising on the use of heat, ask the patient to ensure that the heat source is wrapped in a towel and not applied directly on the skin to prevent burning of the affected area. Hot wax can be used for patients with RA who have painful, swollen and stiff hands. A physiotherapist can show the patient how to apply the wax and provide advice on using the wax safely at home. Cold applications including a bag of peas from the freezer or an ice pack can reduce swelling and pain in a joint. Advice on using ice safely is required. As ice can also burn the skin, the ice needs to be wrapped in a towel before application. The use of ice has been shown to have a beneficial effect on the range of movement, function, knee strength and swelling in knee OA (Brosseau et al. 2003).

7.9.8   Sleep

Pain originating from joint inflammation or joint damage can cause pain at night causing a disturbed sleep pattern. A lack of quality sleep can increase the perception of pain and fatigue making it more difficult to cope with the pain. If sleep disturbance is occurring, then advice on improving sleep, commonly referred to as sleep hygiene, can be given (see Fig. 7.10).

Summary of Main Points
1. A combination of pharmacological and non-pharmacological interventions can be used to provide effective pain management.
2. Pain assessment requires a patient-centred approach that addresses the physical, psychological and social impact of pain.
3. Self-report pain measures are the most valid and reliable means to measure pain.
4. Paracetamol and non-steroidal anti-inflammatory gels are recommended as first line drug treatments for people with osteoarthritis.
5. Older people with arthritis can play an active part in managing their pain by engaging in exercise, pacing and goal setting.

- Develop a sleep routine
- Avoid sleeping in the day
- Increase physical activity
- Only use the bedroom for sleeping avoid other activities such as watching television
- Avoid stimulants such as coffee and alcohol
- Ensure that the bedroom is well ventilated

Fig. 7.10   Sleep hygiene advice

7.10   Self-Assessment

Assessing your own learning and performance needs regarding pain management in the older person. Having read the chapter and undertaken further study, the following are some ideas as to how to relate what you have learnt to your practice:

1. Consider how you currently assess an older person's pain. What actions can you introduce to ensure a patient-centred assessment approach is used.
2. Identify the pain assessment measures currently used in your workplace to assess pain. What are the strengths and limitations of these measures? Which measure would be most effective at helping you understand the impact of pain of all aspects of function?
3. Discuss with your colleagues the safest and most effective drug treatments to use in an older person with joint pain.
4. Discuss with your colleagues the different non-pharmacological approaches that exist to manage pain. Identify a new approach that you could use in your clinical area.

References

Abdilla A, Adams N, Bone M, et al. Guidelines on the management of pain in older people. Age Aging. 2013;42(Suppl 1):i1–i57.
Bellamy N, Buchanan WW, Goldsmith CH, Campbell J, Still LW. Validation study of WOMAC: a health status instrument for measuring clinically important patient relevant outcomes to anti-rheumatic drug therapy in patients with OA of the hip and knee. J Rheumatol. 1988;15(12):1833–40.
Bevers K, Kishino N, Gatchel R. The biopsychosocial model of the assessment, prevention and treatment of chronic pain. US Neurol. 2016;12(2):98–104.
British Pain Society. The assessment of pain in older people, national guidelines. 2007. Accessed via the British Society of Pain website: www.britishpainsociety.org.
Brosseau L, Yonge KA, Robinson V. Thermotherapy for treating OA of the knee. Cochrane Database Syst Rev. 2003;(4):CD004522.
Doherty M, Abhishek A. Osteoarthritis. In: Adebajo A, Dunkley L, editors. ABC of rheumatology. 5th ed. London: BMJ Books, Wiley-Blackwell; 2018. p. P55–60.
Ehde DM, Dillworth T, Turner A. Cognitive behavioral therapy for individuals with chronic pain. Am Psychol. 2014;69(2):153–66.
Fairbank JC, Pynsent P. The Oswestry Disability Index. Spine. 2000;25(22):2940–53.
Fernandes L, Hagaen KB, Bijisma JW, et al. EULAR recommendations for the non-pharmacological core management of hip and knee OA. Ann Rheum Dis. 2013;72:1125–35.
Fransen M, McConnell S, Hernandez-Molina G, Reichenbach S. Exercises for OA of the hip. Cochrane Database Syst Rev. 2009;(3):CD007913.
Garrow AP, Papageorgiou AC, Silman AJ, Thomas E, et al. Development and validation on a questionnaire to assess disability in foot pain. Pain. 2000;85:107–13.
Geenan R, Overmann CL, Christensen R, Asenlof P, et al. EULAR recommendations for the health professional's approach to pain management in inflammatory arthritis and osteoarthritis. Ann Rheum Dis. 2018;77:797–807.
Hudak PL, Amadio RC, Bombardier C. Development of an upper extremity outcome measure: the DASH. Am J Ind Med. 1996;29(6):602–8.
Iverson MD. Managing hip and knee OA with exercise-what is the best prescription. Ther Adv Musculoskelet Care. 2010;2(5):279–90.

Kumar KH, Elavarasi P. Definitions of pain and classification of pain disorders. J Adv Clin Res Insights. 2016;3:87–90.

Laslett L, Jones G. Capsaicin for OA pain. Prog Drug Res. 2014;68:277–91.

Machando G, Maher C, Ferreira PH. Efficacy and safety of paracetamol for spinal pain and OA. Systematic review and meta-analysis of randomised placebo controlled trials. BMJ. 2015;350:h1225.

Melzack R, Wall PD. Pain mechanisms: a new theory. Science. 1965;150(3699):971–9.

Merskey H, Bogduk N. Classification of chronic pain: description of chronic pain syndromes and definition of pain terms. In: Task force on taxonomy of the International Association for the Study of Pain. 2nd ed. Seattle: ISAP Press; 1994.

Mordecai L, Reynolds C, Donaldson LJ, et al. Patterns of regional variation of opioid prescribing in primary care in England: a retrospective observational study. Br J Gen Pract. 2018;68(668):e225–33.

National Institute for Health and Care Excellence. Osteoarthritis: care management. CG 117. 2014. https://www.nice.org.uk/guidance/cg177.

National Institute for Health and Care Excellence. Osteoarthritis: overview. 2017. https://pathways.nice.org.uk/pathways/osteoarthritis

Rannou F, Pelletier JP, Martel-Pelletier J. Efficacy and safety of topical NSAIDs in the management of osteoarthritis. Evidence from real life settings, trials and surveys. Seminar Arthritis Rheum. 2016;45(4 Suppl):S18–21.

Roland M, Fairbank J. The Roland Morris Disability Index and the Oswestry Disability Index. Spine (Phila Pa 1976). 2000;25(24):3115–24.

Sabzwari SR, Qedwai W, Bhanji S. Polypharmacy in the elderly: a cautious trail to tread. J Pak Med Assoc. 2013;63(5):624–7.

Schofield P. The assessment of pain in older people: UK national guidelines. Age Aging. 2018;47:i1–i22. https://doi.org/10.1093/ageing/afx192.

Shakoor N, Lidtke RH, Wimmer MA, et al. Improvement in knee loading after use of specialised footwear for knee OA: results of a 6 month pilot investigation. Arthritis Rheum. 2013;65(5):1282–9.

Sharpe L. Psychological management of chronic pain in patients with rheumatoid arthritis: challenges and solutions. J Pain Res. 2016;9:137–46.

Stannard C. Opioids in the UK, what's the problem? BMJ. 2013;342:f5108.

Tan G, Jensen MP, Thornby JI, Bilel FS. Validation of the BFI for chronic non malignant pain. J Pain. 2004;5(2):133–7.

Tung DL, Raizada SR. Fibromyalgia in the context of RA: a review. Fibromyalgia: Open Access. 2016;1(1):103.

Uthman O, van der Windt D, Jordan J, et al. Exercise for lower limb OA: systematic review incorporating sequential analysis and network meta-analysis. BMJ. 2013;347:f5555.

Vardeh D, Mannion R, Woolf C. Towards a mechanism based approach to pain diagnosis. J Pain. 2016;17(9):50–69.

Wang A. GP pain management: what are the 'Ps' and 'As' of pain management. Aust Fam Physician. 2014;43(8):537–40.

Wheeler AH, Goolkasian P, Baird AC, Darden B. Development of the neck pain and disability scale: item analysis, face and criterion related validity. Spine. 1999;24(13):1290.

Further Reading

Access the International Association for the Study of Pain at https://www.isap-pain.org/ look at the Special Interest Groups (SIG) for musculoskeletal pain and read the fact sheet on evidence-based biopsychosocial treatment of chronic musculoskeletal pain.

Access the pain tool kit at https://www.paintoolkit.org. Look at the resources available for healthcare professionals. Which of these resources could you use to enhance your practice.

Oliver S. Chapter 15: Pharmacological management of pain relief. In: Oxford handbook of musculoskeletal nursing. Oxford: Oxford University Press; 2009.

The Psychological and Social Impact of Arthritis

8

Elizabeth Hale

8.1 Learning Outcomes

Using the text and case studies, at the end of the chapter, the nurse will be able to:

- Identify the signs and symptoms of depression in adults and older adults
- Be familiar with one commonly used measure for depression
- Know the difference between body image and self-image
- Understand how both men and women may respond to changes in body image
- Recognise that sexual relationships continue to be important and signpost patients to information resources
- Identify the key social roles that patients may have in their lives
- Know how to ask patients about different sources of social support and the importance of maintaining valued activities

8.2 Introduction

8.2.1 Considering the 'Biopsychosocial'

The biopsychosocial concept or model (Fig. 8.1) is intended to encompass the range of factors to consider when we think about how health and illness affect the individual or even entire societies. It is literally a coming together of the *biological* (physical health or illness), the *psychological* (mind and behaviour) and the *sociological* (social structures and cultural factors). Although these psychosocial factors

E. Hale (✉)
Department of Rheumatology, The Dudley Group NHS Foundation Trust, Russells Hall Hospital, Dudley, UK
e-mail: Elizabeth.Hale@dgh.nhs.uk

© Springer Nature Switzerland AG 2020
S. Ryan (ed.), *Nursing Older People with Arthritis and other Rheumatological Conditions*, Perspectives in Nursing Management and Care for Older Adults, https://doi.org/10.1007/978-3-030-18012-6_8

Fig. 8.1 The
biopsychosocial model

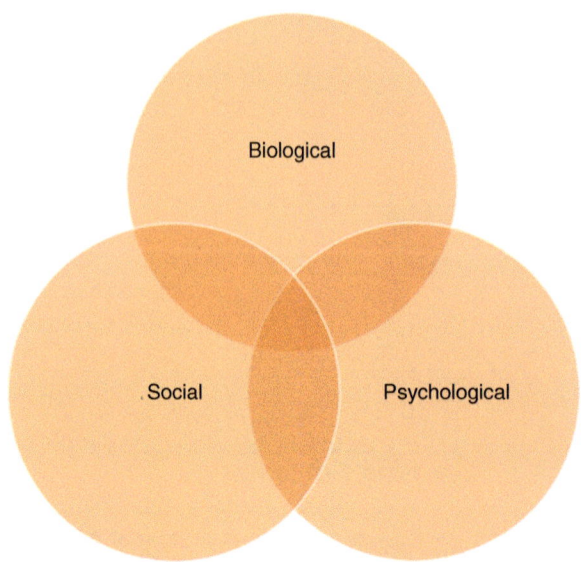

will be discussed separately, it is worth noting that they are often interrelated and impact upon each other. Equally, the psychosocial factors that we will examine are not considerations *exclusive* to the older adult, but are relevant across the lifespan.

Where appropriate, small case studies will be presented. You can use these to assess and develop your knowledge for your own practice.

8.3   Low Mood

In 2018 the World Health Organization (WHO) stated that depression is the leading cause of disability worldwide (World Health Organisation 2018). Additionally, average 'health scores' for people who have depression and chronic physical health conditions are lower, indicating a strong relationship between the two (World Health Organisation 2007).

The relationship between physical health and mental health is complex and bidirectional (it works in both directions). Rheumatic conditions, such as rheumatoid arthritis (RA) and osteoarthritis (OA), present significant challenges for the individual and family to cope with (Matcham et al. 2016; Hampson et al. 1996). Pain (see Chapter 7), fatigue (see Chapter 6), medication and its side effects, changes in work and social roles and decreased mobility may all have an impact upon mood (Matcham et al. 2013). People with RA who also experience depression have been shown to do less well in terms of treatment outcome. The presence of depressive symptoms at the start of biologic treatment has been shown to be associated with 20–40% reduced odds of good treatment response at 1-year follow-up, with reduced improvement in disease activity over time (Matcham et al. 2018).

Individuals who have been formerly depressed *prior* to developing RA have also been observed to fare less well in their ability to cope with symptoms such as pain and may experience a re-occurrence of low mood (Conner et al. 2006). Indeed, levels of depression and anxiety have been reported to be higher than the general population in people with RA and can persist over time and reduce treatment effectiveness and other health outcomes (Matcham et al. 2018).

8.3.1   How Do I Recognise Depression?

The National Institute for Health and Care Excellence (NICE) acknowledges the link between long-term health conditions and the risk of developing depression and offers guidelines for assessment and treatment in adults (NICE 2017). The NICE guidelines follow the criteria laid down by the American Psychiatric Association's Diagnostic and Statistical Manual of Mental Disorders (DSM V) which enables a formal diagnosis of a depressive disorder to be made (American Psychiatric Publishing 2013).

If a patient seems 'low' or mentions that they are 'down' or 'depressed', it is worth investigating further. Ask the following questions:

- During the last month, have you often been bothered by feeling down, depressed or hopeless?
- During the last month, have you often been bothered by having little interest or pleasure in doing things?

We all feel low or miserable from time to time, but it is the *persistence* of symptoms that is particularly key. Try and establish whether symptoms are experienced every day, for most of the day, for at least 2 weeks. If they are, at least *five* other symptoms should *also* be present and mark a notable change to usual functioning in order to indicate a diagnosis of depression:

- Significant weight loss or gain, or significant change in appetite
- Hypersomnia or insomnia nearly every day
- Noticeable (by others) slowing down or agitation
- Fatigue every day
- Feeling worthless or feeling excessively or inappropriately guilty
- Inability to concentrate or being indecisive
- Thoughts of death: suicidal ideation with or without an attempt or plan

If a diagnosis of depression appears indicated, it will be important to establish whether similar symptoms might reasonably be expected due to the nature of the rheumatic condition or as a result of treatment effects. For example, changes in appetite, disrupted sleep patterns and excessive fatigue are all potential features of several rheumatic conditions. Care must be taken to disentangle, where possible, those effects that are due to the physical health of the individual and those that indicate deteriorating psychological wellbeing.

As well as a good 'clinical interview' within the consultation, nurses might find the nine-item Patient Health Questionnaire (PHQ-9, Fig. 8.2) to be a useful self-administered scale for adults, based upon earlier DSM (IV) criteria

Over the last **2 weeks**, how often have you been bothered by any of the following problems? *(Circle one number to indicate your answer)*	Not at all	Several days	More than half the days	Nearly every day
Little interest or pleasure in doing things	0	1	2	3
Feeling down, depressed or hopeless	0	1	2	3
Trouble falling or staying asleep or sleeping too much	0	1	2	3
Feeling tired or having little energy	0	1	2	3
Poor appetite or overeating	0	1	2	3
Feeling bad about yourself – or that you are a failure or have let yourself or family down	0	1	2	3
Trouble concentrating on things, such as reading the newspaper or watching television	0	1	2	3
Moving or speaking so slowly that other people could have noticed? Or the opposite — being so fidgety or restless that you have been moving around a lot more than usual	0	1	2	3
Thoughts that you would be better off dead or hurting yourself in some way	0	1	2	3
Score				

Total score:

Fig. 8.2 The Patient Health Questionnaire 9 (PHQ-9)

Table 8.1 Score interpretation for PHQ-9

PHQ-9 score	Level of depressive symptom severity
0–4	None
5–9	Mild depression
10–14	Moderate depression
15–19	Moderately severe depression
20–27	Severe depression

(Kroenke et al. 2001). Scores indicate both presence and level of severity of a depressive disorder which enable signposting or referral to appropriate services (NICE 2009, 2017).

Scores on the PHQ-9 can range from 0 to 27, with higher scores indicating greater severity of depression (Table 8.1). If three or more questions are unanswered, the PHQ-9 should not be scored. If one or two questions are unanswered, calculate the total of scores answered, multiply by 9, and divide the answer by the number of questions answered (round to nearest whole number).

People who have 'sub-threshold' depression should be monitored or the general practitioner (GP) made aware of the existence of borderline depressive symptoms. If this persists, the GP may offer individual guided self-help based on cognitive behavioural therapy (CBT) which may be via a computerised course (CCBT). Alternatively there may be group-based activities available. Medications using anti-depressant therapies are not advocated at this stage as the risk/benefit ratio is poor (NICE 2009).

8.3.2   Depression in Older Adults

Perhaps contrary to expectations, depression is common in older adults (65 years and older) (Vieira et al. 2014). Older adults, simply by virtue of age, are more likely to have physical health problems, which in turn increase the risk for depression (Pocklington 2017). Estimates suggest 40% of people aged over 65% and 69% of those aged over 85 have a long-term physical illness (Age 2016).

Older age in the rheumatic diseases has been linked to increases in comorbidity and polypharmacy (Treharne et al. 2007). Depression can negatively affect physical disorders and can promote disability by social withdrawal and inactivity (Alexopoulos 2005). The adage 'the less you do, the less you *can* do' is especially relevant for people with rheumatic conditions. Cardiovascular disease risk is elevated in those with RA, and modification of lifestyle factors (diet, exercise, giving up smoking) is something only the individual can commit to (John et al. 2010). Depression and advancing age may make these targets seem insurmountable, and support will be needed to help with this (National Rheumatoid Arthritis Society 2019).

Triggers for an episode of depression may be the death of a loved one, loneliness and isolation, financial worries as well as ill-health. After the age of 65, newly presenting depression is termed 'late-onset' and may be characterised by a slightly different presentation of symptoms than those seen in younger adults. Mood (affect) may not be altered; this has been termed 'depression without sadness' and may mean it is overlooked (Pocklington 2017). Alternatively, physical symptoms may be reported rather than emotional symptoms, and anxiety or agitation may be more prominent. It is important to rule out dementia (vascular or otherwise). In general 'don't know' answers in cognitive testing suggest depression (pseudodementia), whereas speech and word-finding difficulties are linked to dementia (Mueller et al. 2017).

Older adults may also be reluctant to seek help for low mood. The reasons for this can be generational—a 'get on with it' attitude can be a difficult habit to break. Additionally, older adults may perceive depression as a 'weakness' or failure, something to be ashamed of, and they may be disinclined to trouble others with their problems. They may be anxious that admitting to depression might bring a loss of independence and a source of unwelcome interference in their lives.

Cultural factors may prevent openness in help-seeking and the expression of distress (language used and symptoms) may be different. Careful exploration will be required here.

Case Study: Norman

Norman, aged 63, has psoriatic arthritis (PsA), an inflammatory rheumatic condition characterised by inflammation in and around the joints together with the skin condition psoriasis. His treatment has been very effective in improving his psoriasis, such that it hardly troubles him. Norman continues to work full-time in local government

At his outpatient review appointment, his clinical nurse specialist (CNS) Susan notices that he is unshaven and is wearing a 'fleece'-style jacket, T-shirt and casual trousers. Usually he is smartly dressed in shirt, tie and suit trousers, often on his way to work after the appointment

Norman is quieter than usual and does not seem to be his usual conversational self. He has had a recurring chest infection due to his immunosuppression therapy and appears disheartened with treatment as it has been intermittent due to the infections. He comments that further treatment seems a waste of time as nothing seems to help. His inflammatory markers were mildly raised, suggesting there may be PsA disease activity or infection

Susan gently asks Norman how he is feeling about things, and after much prompting, he eventually tells her that he is currently taking sickness absence from work as he was finding it hard to concentrate. He realised he was unusually irritable with junior colleagues and recalled an incident at work when he had shouted at his manager

Norman appeared generally miserable and admitted he wasn't doing much at home except sleeping a lot. His appetite was poor and he had lost weight in the last few weeks. His wife, who accompanied him to the appointment, wondered if he might be depressed as his behaviour was out of character. Norman said he didn't want to trouble Susan with his problems, and said he 'just needed to get on with it'

Self-assessment: What features of Norman's story might Susan consider in helping her to decide whether he is suffering from depression?

8.4   Body Image and Sexual Relationships

Body image is a multidimensional construct made up of attitudes and feelings about one's body, particularly those relating to physical appearance (Jolly et al. 2012). Understandably, self-perceptions about the way we look and present ourselves to the world are very individual and subjective, and they will reflect, to a certain extent, generational, cultural (and sub-cultural) norms and identities.

- *Body image* is often about physical appearance and therefore *externally* located to the body.
- *Self-image* is a related concept and may be more *internally* located and reflect how you feel about yourself as a person.

The relationship between body image and self-image is likely to be bidirectional and can be influenced by the onset of a physical health condition and may affect the way in which people subsequently cope. Difficulties in accepting changes to body image may impact upon self-image and affect mood.

In research with people who have systemic lupus erythematosus (SLE), participants indicated a negative view of their body image, but a positive view of their self-image, locating personal 'worth' within the body (Hale et al. 2015). Women who previously placed greater emphasis on their external appearance found they had to rethink where their 'value' lies:

> Well, well, I cannot put any stock on the outside of my body, because I was, I think, always so vain and always stayed in shape and this and that and everything was perfect. But what's the heart of it is in my heart, you know, that I do feel good about myself. I do know that I am a worthy human being and an honest human being, you know, and I have good morals, and…I don't feel any negative, you know, about myself—quote from Patient 15, aged 57, Hale et al. (2015), p. 1223.

Rheumatic conditions can result in a number of changes to the external appearance. Both the disease process itself and the treatment for it can contribute to this. Depending on the disorder, there may be joint swelling and deformity, changes in posture, gait and movement, skin rashes and lesions, loss of skin pigmentation, scarring and alopecia. Treatment with corticosteroids may result in weight gain, bruising, osteoporosis and a rounding of the face (Cushingoid) resulting in a 'moon-faced' appearance (Hale et al. 2015).

In modern Western society, the concept of attractiveness or beauty carries a value judgement. Attractive people (of any age and particularly when it comes to women) are perceived as being more intelligent, more sociable and of good character and to have better mental health. Attractive people also tend to secure better jobs (Feingold 1992; Davis et al. 2001). In a study with women (mean age 57) who had RA, the desire for hand surgery was motivated by appearance concerns *more than* restoration of physical function (Vamos 1990). Changes to outward appearance due to the onset of physical illness may have far-reaching consequences and can lead to people becoming withdrawn and isolated.

Needing to use visible aids and devices when recommended, such as a walking stick, can be a psychological challenge to overcome. Whilst stability and confidence may be restored with a walking aid, this also means becoming more observable. It has been observed that the body when healthy is *disappeared* (it doesn't require attention); however, when the body becomes unwell, it *dys-appears* (it requires attention and therefore becomes visible) (Leder 1990). Whilst the use of assistive aids is common, it is often equated with older age groups. This means that younger adults face questions about legitimisation 'you're too young to need a walking stick', and older adults may see the aid as a signalling of old age, poor health and disability (Martin et al. 2000).

Much of the research that has been carried out into body image and related concepts has been with women and often with young student populations. However, concerns around body image, self-image and identity are as relevant for men as women and for any age group (Martin et al. 2000; Baker and Gringart 2009).

Interviews with men diagnosed with RA aged between 44 and 75 years revealed they tried to hide their rheumatic condition in public in order to maintain a 'masculine' image, which was equated with strength, independence and 'normality' (Fleury et al. 2017). Women have been observed to use clothing in a deliberate attempt to conceal parts of their bodies they were unhappy with, in order to deflect attention towards the clothes themselves (Hale et al. 2006). There may be genuine concerns about revealing a chronic health condition such as arthritis, fearing judgement from others. Even when external appearance is less affected, the decision to reveal oneself as 'disabled' has been likened to 'coming out' (Swain and Cameron 1999).

8.4.1   Sexual Relationships

Individuals with rheumatic conditions may also face difficulties in sexual relationships (Puchner et al. 2019). Fatigue, depression, swollen, tender or restricted movement in joints; pain; and/or body image concerns due to weight gain or rashes may discourage individuals from intimate relationships leading to sexual dysfunction (Yilmaz 2013). Difficulties are not necessarily related to *severity* of disease (in this case RA) although the number of people experiencing sexual dysfunction, but not seeking help for it, may be underestimated (Puchner et al. 2019). Patients have attributed a lack of sexual intimacy to the breakdown of their relationships, which was linked to the effects of their condition and the medication taken for it (Hale et al. 2015). Older adults may find it easier to 'reorient' their intimacy beyond the physical act of sex if partners are understanding, empathic and accepting of change (Helland et al. 2011). Communication is vital to avoid misunderstandings and conflict. There may be difficulties having conversations with partners about retaining sexual attractiveness, putting strain on relationships (Williams and Barlow 1998).

In healthcare settings nurses are well placed to ask how relationships are faring in the context of the rheumatic condition. Indirect questioning can be useful, becoming more specific if the patient and ideally their partner are open to discussing the subject. A national patient charity in the United Kingdom (UK), Versus *Arthritis*, produced a useful booklet with practical suggestions to help maintain intimacy, such as taking painkillers an hour before sex and taking a warm bath or shower together to ease joint pain (Versus Arthritis 2014).

Healthcare professionals also need to be aware of specific issues that may affect the health and wellbeing of disabled people within the LGBT community. LGBT people experienced a lack of understanding of specific healthcare needs by healthcare staff (Bachmann and Gooch 2017). In certain groups this is even higher, with 62% of trans people experiencing this. Three in five disabled LGBT people have also felt that life was not worth living at some point in the last year. For older adults, or those in rural communities with less access to supportive groups, these issues may place an additional burden upon mental wellbeing and need to be acknowledged.

8.4.2   Assessing Body Image

As body image is a multidimensional construct, formal 'measures' of this have been problematic, and results can be interpreted in different ways dependent upon the socio-demographic variables (such as sex and age) of the people being surveyed. Researchers have highlighted the difficulties posed by questions about body satisfaction as a measure of body image. The item 'I am satisfied with my body' (Baker and Gringart 2009, p. 978) may be answered differently by younger and older people. Older people may relate this to physical wellbeing, whereas younger people may relate it to physical appearance. This means it is unclear what is being measured and interpreted. Physical fitness as a component of body image remains a significant factor in how older men evaluate their bodies (Baker and Gringart 2009).

In clinical practice, a good clinical interview sensitively handled should be able to discriminate what aspects of body image, self-image and identity an individual might be having difficulty with and how this might be related to outcomes such as low mood or social withdrawal.

Case Study: Joanna

Joanna is a married, retired, homemaker aged 65. She is often accompanied to her outpatient appointments by her elder sister Sophie

Joanna has both rheumatoid arthritis and osteoarthritis in her knees. She has had a diagnosis of RA for 18 months and has been managed with disease-modifying anti-rheumatic drugs (DMARDS) so far

Her hands and wrists are swollen today and she walks painfully into the consulting room. Her consultant rheumatologist notices that her blood tests and disease activity score (DAS) show her RA is in a 'flare' or active phase and will probably require an escalation of treatment

Joanna looks distressed and her sister tells the doctor that Joanna 'had a little cry' in the waiting room when she saw that one of the women had some lovely high-heeled shoes. Joanna used to love to dress smartly, and this included fashionable shoes. She can no longer wear most of her old shoes and is struggling to get clothes on and off

Sophie is concerned that Joanna is 'giving up' and becoming withdrawn and isolated. She is refusing to go shopping and prefers to stay at home rather than go to social events as she 'doesn't like people looking at her'. Joanna says that she feels 'old' and tired, and she is worried that her husband of many years will feel differently about her because of the way she looks

Self-assessment: Discuss with a range of colleagues if possible (e.g. doctor, physiotherapist, occupational therapist, podiatrist) what they notice about Joanna's story. What could they offer to support her from their specialist perspective? What could you do?

8.5   Social Roles, Valued Activities and Social Support

Social roles, valued activities and social support are inter-related concepts that impact upon each other.

8.5.1 Social Roles

As members of society we all have a variety of social roles, and we change our behaviour, and possibly our outward appearance, according to the social role we are in. For example, the author is a daughter, mother, spouse, sister, cousin, aunt, friend, colleague, employee, psychologist, teacher and researcher. In all of these roles, certain tasks and behaviours will be expected, although they will vary according to the individual, culture and society.

Social roles are highly valued aspects of our lives, and changes to, or the loss of, these roles due to the onset of a rheumatic condition may be very difficult for both the individual and their families and friends. Qualitative research with men and women with RA (half of whom were aged over 65) indicated that the division of labour within the household often changed, with the spouse taking more responsibility for household tasks (Kristiansen et al. 2012). This was a double-edged sword for the person with RA who was both grateful for the help, but guilty at the extra burden placed on the other by the change in their social role.

Older adults may need extra help from grown-up children, yet find it hard to ask for it, again not wishing to be a 'nuisance'; they may also be uncomfortable with the social role reversal of child caring for parent (Kristiansen et al. 2012). Alternatively, there may be difficulties in getting adult children and grandchildren to understand that extra help is required, as they may be unwilling to accept that a parent is struggling. Both grandparents and parents have also expressed frustration at not being able to 'keep up' with children/grandchildren due to their rheumatic condition, or fulfil caring tasks such as hair brushing and plaiting (Grant et al. 2004; Hale et al. 2009). Changes to pre-arranged plans due to pain or fatigue can make the parent/grandparent feel guilty. This has been expressed as 'I let you down again syndrome' (Barlow et al. 1999). Pain, distress and frustration can also result in angry outbursts at children/grandchildren when they misbehave, causing guilt and regret later (Hale et al. 2009).

8.5.2 Social Support

Social scientists often define 'social support' in terms of the kinds of support people receive from, and provide to, others. People tend to offer three main types of support—emotional, instrumental or 'practical' and informational. *Emotional* support might be talking through a problem with someone and offering a shoulder to cry on; *practical* support might be offering to take someone to a hospital appointment; and *informational* might be the kind of support healthcare practitioners offer to patients about their condition. In order to fulfil certain social roles, people may need to utilise social support in a different way.

Social support is known to provide beneficial effects to both physical and psychological wellbeing (Penninx et al. 1997). This might be because social support has a *direct effect* on health outcomes, or because it acts almost as a *buffer effect* between negative stressful events (like ill-health) and health outcomes (Fig. 8.3).

Fig. 8.3 Direct and buffering effects of social support

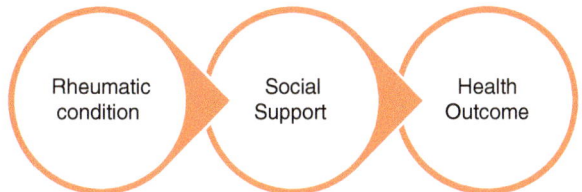

The kind of social support often provided by close relationships from spouses or partners has been shown to provide both positive *and* negative effects on psychological adjustment and physical health outcomes in rheumatic conditions. Lots of support from a spouse has been shown to predict a more active coping style in people with RA (Manne and Zautra 1989), whilst critical and negative remarks resulted in maladaptive coping (a coping strategy that in itself can produce problems, such as excessive drinking).

Where possible, it may be useful to involve spouses and partners in clinical consultations, so that they are well informed about the *impact* of a rheumatic condition as well as the physical processes and treatments. Misunderstandings by loved ones, and underestimations of impact of a rheumatic condition, suggest patients may have difficulties in talking to their families about their needs (Ramos-Remus et al. 2014). The nurse may be a useful 'third party' to ask about levels of understanding and support and facilitate conversations between couples and older children. Men find introducing such conversations difficult, particularly when it comes to receiving emotional support (Fleury et al. 2017). People with established (long-term) RA, who perceived their social support as more helpful, have been shown to experience less fatigue (Treharne et al. 2005).

8.5.3 Valued Activities

The impact of a rheumatic condition may make it difficult for individuals to continue with activities that they formerly highly valued. Pain, fatigue and loss of confidence in ability and appearance can lead to the loss or reduction of employment and hobbies (Kristiansen et al. 2012). Older people may fear ridicule or feel shame at visible physical changes and withdraw from social activities which can lead to isolation and deterioration in psychological wellbeing (Martin et al. 2000). Additionally, the loss of social and emotional support has been linked to cardiovascular symptoms. As people with inflammatory rheumatic disease such as RA have been shown to be at increased risk of cardiovascular events, care should be taken to ensure patients are not becoming socially isolated (Age 2016).

Self-management programmes for people with chronic illnesses provide a specific setting to enhance social support and coping strategies. Often, programmes are built around trying to enhance *self-efficacy*. Self-efficacy relates to an individual's confidence in the ability to carry out tasks even in the face of stress or adversity. Not surprisingly, people with high levels of self-efficacy seem able to cope in more constructive and adaptive ways, and this can improve well-being (Smarr et al. 1997).

Case Study: Jim

Jim is a 55-year-old architect who has had rheumatoid arthritis for 7 years. He has a young son, Paul, aged 7 after re-marrying 10 years ago. He used to enjoy children's football coaching in his spare time; however his RA makes it difficult to run about, so he now takes more of a peripheral role

Jim is treated with a combination of methotrexate and a 'biologic' medication which he has via an infusion at the hospital. He has recently started to work from home 1 day a week as he was finding the car journey to work tiring and was worried that he might not cope. Jim's wife Sandra works full-time as a teacher

Whilst having his infusion, the nurse notices that Jim and his wife seem to be having a quiet argument. After the infusion has finished, the nurse brings Jim a cup of tea and uses the opportunity to chat to the couple

Sandra expresses her frustration at Jim's 'giving up' on many of his 'dad' roles. During a recent snowfall he refused to go sledging with Sandra and his son as he was not confident he could take an active part. He admitted he was worried about what the other parents would think when he did not join in, so he avoided the outing completely. He has no visible signs of RA and thought other dads would assume he was lazy or disinterested

Sandra feels Jim is giving up on valued activities because he is worried about judgement from others. She also feels his working from home is driven by this as well. Sandra complains that she is having to be both 'mum and dad' and is finding this difficult as it impacts on her role as mother and wife. Paul has told her he 'wishes daddy would take him to places again' and wonders 'why daddy doesn't want to play with him anymore'. She wishes Jim would just explain to Paul and other people about his RA

Self-assessment: Are there any local support groups in the community? Have any patient-led groups started in your healthcare setting that you could direct people to?

Summary of Main Points
- There are a range of psychosocial factors that may impact upon health outcomes.
- Depression can have serious outcomes for patients with rheumatic disease and should be a consideration in clinical review.
- Both male and female patients of all ages may experience psychological distress at changes to body image.
- Patients may be reticent in discussing sexual health difficulties, but may appreciate being asked, and signposting to information and other resources.
- A range of social support strategies are important to help patients maintain social roles and valued activities.

8.6   Self-Assessment

Assessing your own learning having read the chapter, the following are some ideas as to how to relate what you have learnt to your practice:

1. List five symptoms that could indicate the presence of depression.
2. Consider how being an older person with arthritis may impact on their social role.
3. Discuss with a colleague how body image might be affected when living with arthritis.
4. Consider developing your own file of resources that you can use to signpost patients and their families to for further help and support.

8.7   Suggested Further Reading/Study

1. Find out more information about the area in which you live or work:
   - Is it predominantly urban or rural?
   - What are the levels of deprivation or affluence?
   - Is it multicultural?
   - What are the rates of disability?
     How might these factors influence psychological and social outcomes in health and wellbeing?
2. Do you know who you would refer someone to if you suspected they had depression?
   - If a patient told you they were suicidal, what would you do?
3. Consider developing your own file of resources that you can readily access to signpost patients and their families to for further help.
   - Be aware of how to refer people in your *local* area and to whom. Have phone contact numbers available and keep them up to date.
   - Resources might also include charities focused on the rheumatic diseases. Some of these are disease specific, whilst some offer generic, evidence-based advice.

References

Age UK. Later life in the United Kingdom. In: Benbow SM, Bhattacharyya S, editors. Older people's mental health and wellbeing. Briefing paper of the British Medical Association. London: BMA; 2016.
Alexopoulos GS. Depression in the elderly. Lancet. 2005;365:1961–70.

American Psychiatric Publishing. Diagnostic and statistical manual of mental disorders. 5th ed. Arlington, VA: American Psychiatric Publishing; 2013.

Bachmann CL, Gooch B. LGBT in Britain: health report. London: Stonewall; 2017.

Baker L, Gringart E. Body image and self-esteem in older adulthood. Ageing Soc. 2009;29:977–95. https://doi.org/10.1017/S0144686X09008721.

Barlow JH, Cullen LA, Foster NE, Harrison K, Wade M. Does arthritis influence perceived ability to fulfill a parenting role? Perceptions of mothers, fathers and grandparents. Patient Educ Couns. 1999;37(2):141–51. https://doi.org/10.1016/s0738-3991(98)00136-0.

Conner TS, Tennen H, Zautra AJ, Affleck G, Armeli S, Fifield J. Coping with rheumatoid arthritis pain in daily life: within-person analyses reveal hidden vulnerability for the formerly depressed. Pain. 2006;126(1–3):198–209. https://doi.org/10.1016/j.pain.2006.06.033.

Davis C, Dionne M, Shuster B. Physical and psychological correlates of appearance orientation. Personal Individ Differ. 2001;30:21–30.

Feingold A. Good-looking people are not what we think. Psychol Bull. 1992;11:304–41.

Fleury CA, Hewlett S, Rodham K, White A, Noddings R, Kirwan JR. "You obviously just have to put on a brave face": a qualitative study of the experiences and coping styles of men with rheumatoid arthritis. Arthritis Care Res. 2017;69(3):330–7. https://doi.org/10.1002/acr.22951.

Grant MI, Foster NE, Wright CC, Barlow JH, Cullen LA. Being a parent or grandparent with back pain, ankylosing spondylitis or rheumatoid arthritis: a descriptive postal survey. Musculoskeletal Care. 2004;2(1):17–28. https://doi.org/10.1002/msc.53.

Hale ED, Treharne GJ, Norton Y, Lyons AC, Douglas KMJ, Erb N, Kitas GD. 'Concealing the evidence': the importance of appearance concerns for patients with systemic lupus erythematosus. Lupus. 2006;15:532–40.

Hale ED, Treharne GJ, Norton Y, Kitas GD. "Are Your Hands Hurting?" Patients' perceptions of the impact of systemic lupus erythematosus on the family unit. Presented at the International Society for critical health psychology biannual conference, Lausanne, Switzerland, July 2009. 2009.

Hale ED, Radvanski DC, Hassett AL. The man-in-the-moon face: a qualitative study of body image, self-image and medication use in systemic lupus erythematosus. Rheumatology. 2015;54(7):1220–5. https://doi.org/10.1093/rheumatology/keu448.

Hampson SE, Glasgow RE, Zeiss AM. Coping with osteoarthritis by older adults. Arthritis Rheum. 1996;9(2):133–41. https://doi.org/10.1002/1529-0131(199604)9:2<133::AID-ANR1790090210>3.0.CO;2-9.

Helland Y, Kjeken I, Steen E, Kvien TK, Hauge M-I, Dagfinrud H. Rheumatic diseases and sexuality: disease impact and self-management strategies. Arthritis Care Res (Hoboken). 2011;63(5):743–50.

John H, Hale ED, Bennett P, Treharne GJ, Carroll D, Kitas GD. Translating patient education theory into practice: developing material to address the cardiovascular education needs of people with rheumatoid arthritis. Patient Educ Couns. 2010;84(1):123–7.

Jolly M, Pickard AS, Mikolaitis RA, Cornejo J, Sequeira W, Cash TF, Block JA. Body image in patients with systemic lupus erythematosus. Int J Behav Med. 2012;19:157–64.

Kristiansen TM, Primdahl J, Antoft R, Hørslev-Petersen K. Everyday life with rheumatoid arthritis and implications for patient education and clinical practice: a focus group study. Musculoskeletal Care. 2012;10:29–38. https://doi.org/10.1002/msc.224.

Kroenke K, Spitzer RL, Williams JB. The PHQ-9: validity of a brief depression severity measure. J Gen Intern Med. 2001;16(9):606–13.

Leder D. The absent body. Chicago, IL: University of Chicago Press; 1990.

Manne SL, Zautra AJ. Spouse criticism and support: their association with coping and psychological adjustment among women with rheumatoid arthritis. J Pers Soc Psychol. 1989;56:608–17.

Martin KA, Leary MR, Rejeski J. Self-presentational concerns in older adults: implications for health and well-being. Basic Appl Soc Psychol. 2000;22(3):169–79. https://doi.org/10.1207/S15324834BASP2203_5.

Matcham F, Rayner L, Steer S, Hotopf M. The prevalence of depression in rheumatoid arthritis: a systematic review and meta-analysis. Rheumatology. 2013;52:2136–48. https://doi.org/10.1093/rheumatology/ket169.

Matcham F, Norton S, Scott DL, Steer, Hotopf M. Symptoms of depression and anxiety predict treatment response and long-term physical health outcomes in rheumatoid arthritis: secondary analysis of a randomized controlled trial. Rheumatology. 2016;55:268–78. https://doi.org/10.1093/rheumatology/kev306.

Matcham F, Davies R, Hotopf M, Kimme HL, Norton S, Steer S, Galloway J. The relationship between depression and biologic treatment response in rheumatoid arthritis: an analysis of the British Society for Rheumatology Biologics Register. Rheumatology. 2018:kex528. https://doi.org/10.1093/rheumatolgy/kex528.

Mueller C, Thompsell A, Harwood D, Bagshaw P, Burns A. Mental health in older people: a practice primer. Redditch/London: NHS England/NHS Improvement; 2017.

National Rheumatoid Arthritis Society. Love your heart. 2019. https://www.nras.org.uk/love-your-heart. Accessed 24 April 2019.

NICE. Depression in adults: recognition and management. National Institute for Health and Care Excellence (NICE). 2009. nice.org.uk/guidance/cg90.

NICE. Depression in adults with a chronic physical health problem: recognition and management. National Institute for Health and Care Excellence (NICE). 2017. nice.org.uk/guidance/cg91.

Penninx B, Van Tilburg T, Deeg D, Kriegsman D, Boeke A, Van Eijk J. Direct and buffer effects of social support and personal coping resources in individuals with arthritis. Soc Sci Med. 1997;44(3):393–402.

Pocklington C. Depression in older adults. Br J Med Pract. 2017;10(1):a1007.

Puchner R, Sautner J, Gruber J, Bragagna E, Trenkler A, Lang G, Eberl G, Alkin A, Pieringer H. High burden of sexual dysfunction in female patients with rheumatoid arthritis: results of a cross-sectional study. J Rheumatol. 2019;46(1):19–26. https://doi.org/10.3899/jrheum.171287.

Ramos-Remus C, Castillo-Ortiz J, Sandoval-Castro C, Paez-Agraz F, Sanchez-Ortiz A, Aceves-Avila F. Divergent perceptions in health-related quality of life between family members and patients with rheumatoid arthritis, systemic lupus erythematosus, and ankylosing spondylitis. Rheumatol Int. 2014;34:1743–9. https://doi.org/10.1007/s00296-014-3044-9.

Smarr KL, Parker JC, Wright GE, Stucky-Ropp R, Buckelew SP, Hoffman RW, O'Sullivan FX, Hewett JE. The importance of enhancing self-efficacy in rheumatoid arthritis. Arthritis Care Res. 1997;10(1):18–26.

Swain J, Cameron C. Unless otherwise stated: discourses of labelling and identity in coming out. In: Corker M, French S, editors. Disability discourse. Buckingham: Open University Press; 1999. p. 68–78.

Treharne GJ, Kitas GD, Lyons AC, Booth DA. Well-being in rheumatoid arthritis: the effects of disease duration and psychosocial factors. J Health Psychol. 2005;10(3):457–74. https://doi.org/10.1177/1359105305051416.

Treharne GJ, Douglas KMJ, Iwasko J, Panoulas VF, Hale ED, Mitton DL, Piper H, Erb N, Kitas GD. Polypharmacy among people with rheumatoid arthritis: the role of age, disease duration and comorbidity. Musculoskeletal Care. 2007;5(4):175–90. https://doi.org/10.1002/msc.112.

Vamos M. Body image in rheumatoid arthritis: the relevance of hand appearance to desire for surgery. Br J Med Psychol. 1990;63:267–77.

Versus Arthritis. Sex and arthritis. Chesterfield: Arthritis Research UK; 2014. https://www.versusarthritis.org/about-arthritis/living-with-arthritis/sex-and-relationships/. Accessed 24 April 2019.

Vieira ER, Brown E, Raue P. Depression in older adults: screening and referral. J Geriatr Phys Ther. 2014;37:24–30. https://doi.org/10.1519/JPT.0b013e31828df26f.

Williams B, Barlow JH. Falling out with my shadow: lay perceptions of the body in the context of arthritis. In: Nettleton S, Watson J, editors. The body in everyday life. London: Routledge; 1998.

World Health Organisation: Geneva, Switzerland, World Health Statistics 2007. Mental illness: depression worsens the health of people with chronic illness. 2007. p. 16. www.who.int/whosis/whostat2007.pdf.

World Health Organisation: Geneva, Switzerland. Depression. 2018. See https://www.who.int/news-room/fact-sheets/detail/depression. Accessed 17 Apr 2019.

Yilmaz H. The association between rheumatoid arthritis and women's sexual dysfunction. Int J Phys Med Rehabil. 2013;1(2):115. https://doi.org/10.4172/2329-9096.1000115.

Drug Therapy

9

Jill Bloxham

9.1 Learning Outcomes

At the end of the chapter, the nurse will be able to:

1. Describe the pharmacological treatment for older people with an arthritic condition
2. Understand the basic mode of action of different treatments used
3. Understand when it is appropriate to use different treatments
4. Explain the potential adverse events of different medications
5. Identify the concerns of using medications in the older person with an arthritic condition

9.2 Introduction

9.2.1 Pharmacological Management of Arthritis

The aim of medical management in people with arthritis is to reduce inflammation and the symptoms of pain, swelling, stiffness and fatigue and to slow or halt disease progression where possible. To protect against the risk of damage to joints, bones and other organs of the body caused by uncontrolled disease. In addition a key aim is to enable the person to lead a normal life with minimal impact on their home life, work, family and leisure activities. A combination of medication is usually required to achieve optimum disease control and satisfactory patient reported outcomes and,

J. Bloxham (✉)
Cambridge University Hospitals NHS Foundation Trust, Cambridge, UK
e-mail: Jill.bloxham@addenbrookes.nhs.uk

© Springer Nature Switzerland AG 2020
S. Ryan (ed.), *Nursing Older People with Arthritis and other Rheumatological Conditions*, Perspectives in Nursing Management and Care for Older Adults,
https://doi.org/10.1007/978-3-030-18012-6_9

129

as not everyone's disease is exactly the same, different people may be started on different drug regimes.

The recommended treatment paradigm for inflammatory arthritis, such as rheumatoid arthritis (RA), has changed significantly in recent years. The introduction of so-called biologic agents has greatly improved outcomes for many people of all ages with inflammatory arthritis (Scott 2002). In order to minimise the likelihood of joint damage, early medical intervention is advocated using disease-modifying medication as first-line treatment alongside medications to treat the pain and stiffness (Emery et al. 2002). A 'treat-to-target' approach is advocated for the management of early inflammatory disease (Smolen et al. 2016), the main 'target' being remission or at least low disease activity. Disease activity is measured by rheumatology health professionals using a disease activity score (DAS) referred to as DAS28, which defines low to severe disease activity. A person's disease activity and response to medications is frequently monitored in order that therapy can be tailored and adapted for the individual person's needs.

In addition, the discovery of some disease-specific biomarkers has increased understanding of the underlying pathogenesis of disease. These biomarkers can help identify disease risk and predict prognosis, target therapy more specifically and assess response to treatment (Robinson and Mao 2016).

9.2.2 Pharmacokinetics and Pharmacodynamics in the Older Person

It is pertinent to consider that most drug studies exclude people over the age of 70 years; therefore, there is very little evidence available to support the safe use of drug treatment in this age group.

However, as age increases, a combination of physiological factors, such as increasing body fat, reduced muscle mass and reduction in fluid balance, can alter drug absorption, distribution, metabolism and excretion. These changes may result in differences in effectiveness and toxicity in the older person (Fine 2012; McCleane 2007). Increasing age is also associated with reduction in hepatic and renal function. Reduced liver function may result in increased plasma concentration and bioavailability of some drugs, such as opioid analgesics. Reduced renal function can increase the half-life (the time it takes for the amount of drug in your body to be reduced by half) of drugs that are normally excreted through the kidneys. Therefore drug doses may need to be lower in older people (Fine 2012). Comorbid conditions and polypharmacy also need to be considered (Stannard and Booth 2004).

In addition, there is a greater likelihood that the older person with arthritis may have some sensory impairment, memory difficulties, limited social support and difficulty accessing treatment. Functional difficulties, such as inability to open medicine packaging, are common in people with arthritis (McCleane 2007). All these factors that accompany ageing are important to consider when making choices about medical management.

9.3   Analgesia

Pain affecting the joints is a primary symptom for people with all rheumatological conditions including RA, osteoarthritis (OA) and gout. Analgesics are often used in combination with non-steroidal anti-inflammatory drugs (NSAIDs) and disease-modifying anti-rheumatic drugs (DMARDs).

Treatment decisions can be complicated for people with arthritis who often require a long-term pain management regime because analgesics that are effective for acute pain are inappropriate for long-term use (van Laar et al. 2012). In addition, the rationale for prescribing painkilling medication in the older person can be complex due to the varied ways that drugs are absorbed, distributed, metabolised and excreted, and variability in analgesic response.

Drugs for managing pain can be divided into three categories: non-opioid, opioid and adjuvant therapies. This section will list the categories of pain-relieving medication and their use in older people.

9.3.1   Non-opioid Analgesics

This group of painkilling drugs includes paracetamol (acetaminophen) and aspirin. It also includes other NSAIDs which will be discussed in a separate section. These drugs are recommended as the first step in the World Health Organization analgesia ladder (WHO 1986).They exert analgesic action both centrally, by preventing the brain from sending signals to the nervous system, and peripherally, when the mechanism of action is outside of the central nervous system. They do not induce tolerance, which is when the person no longer responds to the drug in the way that they did initially, or dependence. They all can be given orally and can be used in addition to opioid analgesic medications.

Paracetamol is the most widely used non-opioid analgesic due to its efficacy and good safety profile (National Institute for Health and Care Excellence 2014). It is used for mild to moderate pain and is recommended for first-line pain relief for OA (National Institute for Health and Care Excellence 2014). When cells are damaged or inflamed, the chemical mediator prostaglandin is released. As discussed in Chapter 7, the mode of action is not fully understood, but paracetamol acts centrally to inhibit cyclo-oxygenase and nitric oxide synthase in the brain which reduces the production of prostaglandins (Stannard and Booth 2004). Paracetamol is absorbed in the upper gastrointestinal (GI) tract and is metabolised in the liver.

Side effects are usually mild and may include constipation. Normally it is considered to be a very safe drug with recommended doses, being 1 gram every 6 hours; however, adverse effects on the renal, GI, hepatic and cardiovascular systems are known and are dose related. Paracetamol does have some peripheral prostaglandin inhibition and there is growing evidence to associate it with GI bleeding especially when used in combination with an NSAID (Hinz and Brune 2012). Co-prescribing with warfarin should be avoided as it can prolong the international normalised ratio (Calderia et al. 2015). In addition caution and close surveillance is required in the elderly, the poorly nourished and those with chronic liver disease who are more at risk of developing liver toxicity (Stannard and Booth 2004).

9.3.2 Compound Analgesics

Compound analgesics combine a non-opioid with an opioid agent. These drugs can be used to bridge the gap between the two strengths of analgesia. Co-codamol is a combination of paracetamol and codeine phosphate which is widely used to treat mild to moderate arthritic pain. People taking co-codamol should be aware that it contains the maximum dose of paracetamol; therefore, additional paracetamol should not be taken.

9.3.3 Opioid Drugs

Opioid drugs are mainly inhibitory in their action; they bind to opioid receptors and mimic the actions of naturally occurring endogenous opioid peptides resulting in reduced transmission of nociceptive impulses.

Opioid drugs can be classified by their strength. Weaker opioid drugs, such as codeine, tramadol, dihydrocodeine and meptazinol, can be used for mild to moderate arthritic pain relief and are particularly effective for acute flares of arthritis. Tramadol, which is taken orally, is a weak centrally acting opioid that inhibits neuronal reuptake of serotonin. Tramadol has been shown to decrease pain intensity in people with OA and to improve function (Cepeda et al. 2006). Recommended dosing should not exceed 400 mg/day and should be reduced or closely supervised in older patients ($\geq$75 years) (van Laar et al. 2012).

Stronger opioid analgesics include buprenorphine and these may be cautiously recommended for people with arthritis whose quality of life is affected by moderate to severe pain and when other medications and non-pharmacological interventions have been ineffective (National Institute for Health and Care Excellence 2014; Simon et al. 2002; Furlan et al. 2006). Because of concerns about possible dependency and addiction from prolonged use, people who use this group of drugs to manage chronic pain, that is sometimes associated with arthritis, should be carefully monitored by a pain specialist.

Overall, long-term use of opioids for chronic conditions is not recommended particularly as they are usually only effective for 12–18 weeks. In addition all opioid analgesics are associated with the following side effects (Stannard 2013) which are more common in the elderly and largely limit their use:

- Nausea and vomiting
- Constipation
- Drowsiness
- Impaired cognition
- Respiratory depression (Fine 2012)

The safety and effectiveness of opioids use has not been evaluated in the older population (American Geriatrics Society Panel on the Pharmacological Management of Persistent Pain in older Persons 2009). Therefore, for this group of people, it is recommended that opioid drugs are used in reduced doses or as low-dose transdermal treatment, such as buprenorphine patches, and close supervision is needed (Furlan et al. 2006).

9.3.4 Adjuvant Therapies

Although they are not considered to be front-line analgesic agents, this group of drugs include antidepressant and anti-epileptic drugs that may be used alone or in combination with analgesic drugs. Anti-depressants have an additional antinociceptive action at low dose and are mainly indicated for neuropathic pain resulting from injury to the nervous system. Tricyclic antidepressants, such as amitriptyline, which inhibit the reuptake of noradrenaline and serotonin, are thought to be the most effective. Amitriptyline can have beneficial effects in people with fibromyalgia to help sleep and relieve pain. It can also be helpful for chronic pain and back pain. Modest effects have been noted in RA (Frank et al. 1988) although its antidepressant effect may play a more important role in pain modification in people with inflammatory disease. However, this group of drugs can have a wide variety of unwanted effects on the central nervous system particularly in the older person (Furukawa et al. 2002). Adverse effects which limit their use include drowsiness, incoordination and dizziness, and particular caution is needed when considering use in those who are more likely to experience side effects.

9.3.5 Topical Analgesics

Capsaicin is a topical treatment that can be used, as an adjunct to other treatments, for the management of pain in hand and knee OA (National Institute for Health and Care Excellence 2014). It has a moderate analgesic effect for up to 20 weeks; however, it may take up to 4 weeks to be fully effective. Capsaicin is generally well tolerated, but users are advised not to rub their eyes, take a bath or put their hands in hot water after use as this leads to an unpleasant burning sensation.

9.4 Non-steroidal Anti-Inflammatory Drugs (NSAIDs)

NSAIDs are an integral part of the therapeutic management of common inflammatory conditions including rheumatoid arthritis (NICE 2009; Luqmani et al. 2006). They may also be used in the management of gout and OA (National Institute for Health and Care Excellence 2014). The two main actions of NSAIDs are to provide analgesia and reduce the following symptoms of inflammation:

- Pain
- Swelling
- Stiffness
- Warmth

The mechanism of action of NSAIDs is complex. Prostaglandins are fatty acids that provoke the inflammatory response. Cyclo-oxygenase (COX) is an enzyme that enables the production of prostaglandin. NSAIDs act to suppress prostaglandin synthesis by inhibiting cyclo-oxygenase. The two forms of cyclo-oxygenase are referred to as COX-1 and COX-2.

There are two distinct categories of NSAID which are classified by their chemical structure:

1. Non-selective or conventional NSAIDs which block COX-1 and COX-2:
   • Ibuprofen
   • Diclofenac
   • Naproxen
   • Meloxicam
   • Etodolac
2. Selective or COX-2 inhibitors which selectively inhibit COX-2:
   • Celecoxib
   • Etoricoxib

NSAIDs are most commonly administered orally where they are absorbed from the GI tract, metabolised by the liver and excreted in the urine. Relief of pain and stiffness is felt soon after starting and with continued treatment. Oral NSAIDs may be considered when paracetamol is not effective; however, they are not very potent painkillers for OA and discontinuation rates are high (40–50% at 2 months).

NSAIDs are also available in topical, suppository and intramuscular injection preparations. Topical NSAIDs, which are available as creams, sprays and gels, are strongly recommended before oral NSAIDs for pain relief in hand and knee OA (National Institute for Health and Care Excellence 2014; Hochberg et al. 2012). They provide moderate pain relief without the side effects associated with oral preparations and have been shown to be as effective as oral NSAIDs (Rannou et al. 2016).

All NSAIDs have similar analgesic effects but vary in their potential toxicity and side effects. The side effects can affect many organs in the body as shown in Table 9.1. This table also describes why the side effects occur and recommendations to manage the unwanted effects.

More serious adverse, and potentially life-threatening, events associated with the NSAID use are GI ulceration; cardiovascular events, including heart failure; and renal failure placing some older people at increased risk. People over 60 years have a threefold risk of developing GI complications than younger people (Fine and Herr 2009). Studies have also demonstrated that people over 55 years taking concomitant diuretics are twice as likely to be admitted at hospital with serious congestive cardiac failure (Heerdink et al. 1998). This risk of developing cardiac failure increases further in patients taking aspirin. Oral NSAID use should therefore be avoided in people who already have comorbidities or who have an increased risk of developing gastrointestinal, renal or cardiovascular disease and topical treatments may be the preferred choice. Warfarin is one of the many drugs that are contraindicated for use with NSAIDs.

Table 9.1 NSAID side effects

Organ	Side effect symptoms	Mechanism	Recommendations
GI tract	• Nausea • Vomiting • Dyspepsia • Pain • Gastric ulceration	• COX-1 also has a gastro-protective function; therefore, inhibition of COX-1 by use of non-selective NSAIDs can cause serious gastrointestinal disturbance	• COX-2 inhibitors are considered to be safer than non-selective NSAIDs for people who have experienced gastrointestinal effects • Try topical and suppository preparations • Should always be taken with food • Never exceed maximum dose • Concomitant use of a proton pump inhibitor, such as omeprazole • Stop NSAID use if gastric ulceration occurs
Kidneys	• Hypertension • Oedema	• Reduced renal blood flow • Increased likelihood with advancing age	• Check blood pressure regularly in the elderly • Reduce the NSAID dose
Skin	• Rash • Itching • Photosensitivity • Urticaria	• Allergic reaction	• Try alternative NSAID
Blood	• Anaemia • Prolonged bleeding • Thrombocytopenia	• Gastric ulceration and associated gastric bleeding • Inhibition of platelet agranulocytosis	• Stop NSAID • Contraindicated with warfarin
Central nervous system	• Memory loss • Poor concentration • Dizziness • Headaches	• Nervous system sensitivity to drugs increases with ageing	• Reduce dose • Try alternative NSAID • Stop NSAID
Lungs	• Breathlessness • Bronchospasm and increased incidents of attacks in asthma sufferers	• Inhibition of cyclo-oxygenase	• Reduce dose • Try alternative NSAID • Stop NSAID

Long-term use of NSAIDs is also associated with these potentially serious adverse effects. The British National Formulary therefore recommends that treatment is offered at the lowest dose for the shortest possible time with regular review to monitor for adverse events and risk factors (British National Formulary 76 2018–2019).

9.5   Disease-Modifying Anti-Rheumatic Drugs (DMARDs)

DMARDs constitute the backbone of pharmacological treatment and are considered the first step in the management of inflammatory arthritis such as RA. The term 'disease-modifying' refers to any drug that prevents or retards the progression of joint damage (erosions and joint narrowing) which commonly occurs in inflammatory arthritis. DMARDs are a varied group of compounds with different pharmacokinetic and biochemical properties that affect a range of cellular targets to suppress the body's immune system. They modify the underlying disease process rather than treating the symptoms and are therefore only beneficial in auto-immune diseases and are not used to treat conditions such as OA.

DMARDs should be started in patients as soon as possible after diagnosis (Luqmani et al. 2006), ideally within 3 months (NICE 2009), to suppress disease activity and prevent disability (Smolen et al. 2017a). Because of their complexity, all DMARDs are initiated by a specialist in the management of rheumatic disease (Ledingham et al. 2017). DMARDs are potentially potent and require long-term safety monitoring. They have a risk of serious adverse events including severe infection, neutropenia (abnormally few neutrophils in the blood leading to increased susceptibility to infection) and liver toxicity. Because of their immunosuppressing effect, people taking DMARDs are advised to have the seasonal flu and pneumococcal vaccination (Ledingham et al. 2017). In addition, live vaccines, such as yellow fever, should be avoided with most DMARDs.

When making therapeutic decisions for DMARD treatment, several factors need to be considered, including the presence of comorbidities, drug interactions and patient preference. Patient involvement and education is essential (Ledingham et al. 2017) (see Chapter 12) and should include the following information:

- Explanation of the decision to commence a DMARD
- Dose and frequency
- Method of administration
- Possible side effects
- Monitoring requirements
- Time until expected benefit
- Potential serious adverse effects
- How to seek advice

Once started, regular monitoring, re-evaluation of disease activity and possible dose adjustment or change of treatment regime are needed (Luqmani et al. 2006).

There are three categories of DMARD: traditional DMARDs, synthetic targeted DMARDs and biologic DMARDs.

9.5.1 Traditional DMARDs

The most commonly used drugs in this category are:

- Methotrexate
- Hydroxychloroquine
- Sulfasalazine
- Leflunomide

Traditional DMARDs are long-term treatment that can be used alone as mono-therapy or in combination with another drug in the same group, and they are typically used alongside NSAIDs and/or analgesic drugs. Their effect is not noticed for up to 12 weeks.

Before starting DMARDs an assessment of risk must be carried out; this usually includes laboratory tests to check full blood count, liver and renal function tests. A test for inflammatory markers in the blood, such as erythrocyte sedimentation rate, will normally be performed to provide a baseline by which efficacy can be measured. For people starting methotrexate and leflunomide, a baseline chest X-ray is also required as these drugs can cause chest symptoms. After initiation, the specialist team will monitor people closely for the first 2–3 months of treatment. Once a person is on a stable drug dose, less frequent blood monitoring is recommended (Ledingham et al. 2017) which may be carried out in primary care under the supervision of the specialist team. If there are abnormalities, guidance is available on when the drugs should be temporarily stopped (Ledingham et al. 2017). People taking DMARDs are usually given a patient-held booklet to record their blood results.

Although there is limited data comparing older and younger people on DMARDs (Veena et al. 2006), differences in efficacy and withdrawal rates due to adverse reactions of traditional DMARDs, including methotrexate and sulfasalazine, are not significantly different in older people (Hirshberg et al. 2002).

9.5.1.1 Methotrexate

Methotrexate is the first choice or 'anchor' DMARD for RA (Smolen et al. 2017a), used either as mono-therapy or in combination with another DMARD such as sulfasalazine.

Methotrexate is a folate antagonist and is classified as a cytotoxic drug. Anti-folate agents slow down the production of blood cells and inhibit connective cell tissue division. Methotrexate is administered weekly either orally, usually as tablets, or parenterally in either a subcutaneous or intramuscular injection. The oral route is most frequently used, but injections may be favoured if there is inadequate clinical response or GI side effects with oral methotrexate. Dose escalation regimes and monitoring schedules vary slightly between different centres, but doses used range from 10 to 25 mg weekly according to tolerability and efficacy. Methotrexate is prescribed with weekly folic acid to reduce GI and mucosal side effects as well as to reduce the risk of serious adverse effects, such as over-suppression of white blood cells and liver toxicity. It is recommended that at least 5 mg folic acid is given once weekly, taken on a different day to methotrexate (Ledingham et al. 2017).

Some people treated with methotrexate will experience adverse reactions. Minor side effects or toxicity can usually be managed without stopping the drug by omitting 1–2 doses. Predisposing factors for toxicity are long exposure, high doses, hypoalbuminaemia, renal insufficiency, viral or alcoholic hepatitis, concomitant use of other anti-folate drugs and advanced age. Therefore, in older people and depending on the presence of comorbidities or co-medication which may interact with methotrexate, slower dose increase or lower maintenance doses are considered.

Taking over-the-counter herbal remedies and some antibiotics (trimethoprim and co-trimoxazole) with methotrexate is not recommended as these can interact with methotrexate. In addition, alcohol consumption should be limited to less than 14 units a week spread over the week, as both methotrexate and alcohol are metabolised in the liver increasing the risk of hepatic toxicity. Pulmonary toxicity may be a problem in RA and patients are advised to seek immediate medical advice if they become breathless with a cough. Methotrexate should be discontinued if pneumonitis is suspected. Caution is also recommended in patients with hepatic impairment as methotrexate clearance will be decreased, increasing the risk of toxicity (Bressolle et al. 1998).

9.5.1.2 Sulfasalazine

Sulfasalazine can be taken as single DMARD treatment, but it is frequently combined with methotrexate. In the gut sulfasalazine is broken down into two parts, a sulphonamide antibiotic and a second component that acts to reduce the process driving inflammation in addition to suppressing the over active immune system. It is available as a liquid medicine, but is most frequently taken in tablet form. The daily dose is built up over 4 weeks from 500 mg daily to a usual maintenance dose of 1 g twice daily. Alcohol can be consumed in moderation. Sulfasalazine has been found to be equally effective in all ages, and there is no significant increase in frequency or nature of side effects with advancing age (Wilkieson et al. 1993).

9.5.1.3 Hydroxychloroquine

Hydroxychloroquine is a treatment for malaria, but has also been shown to be effective for treating mild inflammatory arthritis. In more severe disease it may be used in combination with another DMARD like methotrexate. It is only available as a 200 mg tablet and the dose may vary between 200 and 400 mg daily. When used as mono-therapy, no regular blood monitoring is required. Caution is needed in people with eye conditions due to the rare risk of associated retinal damage. Ophthalmology screening is recommended before the drug is started and annual visual checks are recommended (Ledingham et al. 2017).

9.5.1.4 Leflunomide

Unlike other DMARDs in this group, leflunomide was developed specifically to treat inflammatory arthritis. It is available in tablet form as 10, 15 or 20 mg tablets taken daily. Leflunomide can stay in the body for up to a year after stopping it;

Table 9.2 Traditional DMARDs

DMARD	Maintenance dose	Commonly occurring side effects
Methotrexate	10–25 mg weekly	• Nausea, loss of appetite, vomiting, diarrhoea • Mouth ulcers • Skin rash • Hair thinning • Headaches
Sulfasalazine	1–1.5 g twice daily	• Skin rash/itching • Nausea • Headache • Dizziness • Diarrhoea • Tinnitus • Yellow discolouration of urine
Leflunomide	10–20 mg daily	• Diarrhoea • Hypertension • Skin reaction • Numbness and tingling in hands and feet
Hydroxychloroquine	200–400 mg daily	• Abdominal cramps, loss of appetite, nausea • Rash • Headache • Visual changes-blurring

therefore, in some circumstances, such as adverse reactions, wash-out with cholestyramine may be required. Leflunomide can be hypertensive; therefore, regular blood pressure monitoring is advised alongside the regular blood monitoring.

Table 9.2 lists the most common side effects experienced with these drugs.

9.5.2 Targeted Synthetic DMARDs

Janus kinases (Jak) inhibitors are the newest generation of drugs for inflammatory arthritis. Unlike the conventional DMARDs, these agents offer a targeted approach for the management of inflammatory arthritis.

Two Jak inhibitors, tofacitinib and baricitinib, have recently undergone extensive clinical trials and have been approved for use in the UK (NICE 2017a, b). They have been shown to have similar benefit as anti-tumour necrosis factor (anti-TNF) drugs (Keystone et al. 2017) and are recommended by NICE for the 'treatment of moderate to severe active rheumatoid arthritis in adult patients who have responded inadequately to, or who are intolerant to, one or more disease-modifying anti-rheumatic drugs' (NICE 2017b). They can be used as mono-therapy or in combination with methotrexate.

Because they compromise of small molecules, unlike biologic drugs, they can be taken orally. Baricitinib is taken as a daily 4 mg tablet. However, a maintenance dose of 2 mg once daily is appropriate for patients aged 75 years and over and people with chronic or recurrent infections. The recommended maintenance dose of tofacitinib is 5 mg twice daily or 5 mg once daily in people with severe renal impairment.

Jak inhibitors are usually effective within the first few weeks. Common side effects include:

- Nausea
- GI discomfort
- Diarrhoea
- Breathlessness and cough
- Fever
- Joint pain

It is thought that a rare complication of tofacitinib specifically is deep vein thrombosis. Jak inhibitors should be temporarily stopped if a person develops a serious infection until the infection is controlled. Prescribing caution is used in people with repeated or chronic infections, cancer, stomach ulcers, heart problems including hypertension and hypercholesterolemia and lung, renal and liver conditions. These concerns are likely to limit the use of Jak inhibitors in people of advancing age.

9.5.3   Biologic DMARDs

The use of biologic therapies has transformed the management of inflammatory arthritis with a targeted approach that offers an increasingly achievable goal of disease remission. Biological DMARDs, usually in combination with methotrexate, are recommended for people with severe inflammatory arthritis who have not responded to intensive treatment with combinations of conventional DMARDs (NICE 2016).

Cytokines, such as tumour necrosis factor alpha (TNF-α) and interleukin-1 (IL-1), are cell signalling molecules responsible for causing and maintaining the inflammation that damages bone, cartilage and soft tissue. Specific immunoglobulins that block or alter these pro-inflammatory cytokines have been developed and are referred to as biologic drugs. Different biologic drugs target different levels of the auto-immune system and are highly effective in treating RA.

Biologic drugs are made in living cells and comprise large numbers of atoms. As they are very large molecules, they cannot be taken orally and are either given by self-administered subcutaneous injection, usually via an auto-injector, or by IV infusion (see Table 9.3).

Biologic drugs are expensive and not every drug works for every patient. Therefore eligibility criteria and treatment pathways have been developed to guide clinicians through the choices (Deighton et al. 2010; Holroyd et al. 2019).

Common side effects include:

(a) Anti-TNF drugs
   - Injection site skin rash
   - Abdominal pain and nausea
   - Fever
   - Headache

Table 9.3 Biologic drugs

Target cells of the immune system	Biologic drug	Route		Frequency
		IV infusion	Subcutaneous injection	
TNF-α (anti-TNF)	Infliximab	√		Every 6–8 weeks
	Etanercept		√	Once weekly
	Adalimumab		√	Every 2 weeks
	Certolizumab pegol		√	Every 2 weeks
	Golimumab		√	Once monthly
IL-6	Tocilizumab	√	√	Once monthly infusion or once weekly injection
	Sarilumab		√	Every 2 weeks
B-cells	Rituximab	√		×2, 2 weeks apart every 6–12 months
T-cells	Abatacept	√	√	Once monthly infusion or once weekly injection
IL-12/IL-23	Ustekinumab		√	Every 3 months
IL-17A	Secukinumab		√	Once monthly

(b) Other biologic drugs
- Abdominal pain
- Diarrhoea
- Mouth ulcers
- Dizziness
- Fatigue
- Hypertension
- Upper respiratory tract infections

These drugs are not without their potential risks and careful screening before commencement and on-going monitoring by the specialist team is essential. Rare, but serious, risks are associated with different drugs within this group including possible reactivation of tuberculosis, demyelinating disease and diverticulitis. All biologic drugs carry an increased risk of serious infection (Singh et al. 2015) and anyone taking these drugs is advised to stop the drug whilst they are on antibiotic treatment. Patients will also be given specific advice if requiring surgery. Anti-TNF drugs can be used regardless of age (Fleiscmann et al. 2003) and older people treated with anti-TNF are not at greater risk of developing serious infections (Schneeweiss et al. 2007). Although there is no conclusive evidence of an increased risk of some cancers, vigilance is required and biologic therapies are not commenced in people who have a malignancy (Holroyd et al. 2019).

9.6   Corticosteroids

Corticosteroids, usually known as steroids, have been shown to be effective at reducing inflammation in RA (Criswell et al. 2004) and they have an important role in the management of early inflammatory arthritis for symptom relief before

DMARDs are effective. Studies have shown that patients treated early in their condition will continue to benefit from reduced joint damage many years later, even after the glucocorticoids have been stopped (Luqmani et al. 2006). Steroids can also be effective used alongside other therapies in poorly controlled or aggressive disease or during disease flares. In addition to their benefit for inflammatory arthritis, the National Institute for Health and Care Excellence (NICE) recommends that intra-articular steroids can be used as an adjunct to core treatments, for the relief of pain in OA (National Institute for Health and Care Excellence 2014).

Cortisone and hydrocortisone are naturally occurring chemicals which control metabolism and are produced from the adrenal glands. Synthetic corticosteroids, such as prednisolone, reduce inflammation by binding to intercellular receptors to block particular cytokines and thereby inhibiting T-cell activation and proliferation.

Steroids are effective within a few days and a larger dose, 25 mg daily for example, will have a quicker and larger effect. In some people steroids can also provide a 'sense of well-being' particularly when given in large doses although the reason for this effect is not understood.

They can be administered via different routes and doses as detailed in Table 9.4.

Table 9.4 Steroids

Steroid drug	Route	Recommendations/cautions
Prednisolone (5–20 mg)	Orally	• The optimum dose is the lowest that induces a response • A reducing dose regime is required depending on the dose and length of course • The carrying of a steroid card with information detailing the treatment regime is recommended
Methylprednisolone (Depo-Medrone) (40–120 mg)	Intramuscularly	• Deep intramuscular injection • Can be given as 'bridging' therapy to help control symptoms before DMARDs are effective or to control disease flares
Methylprednisolone (10–80 mg) Triamcinolone (10–40 mg)	Intra-articularly or soft tissue	• Can be effective for up to 3 months • One-third of injections are ineffective • Need to rest for 24–48 h after • Contraindications include local infection, fracture, anticoagulation therapy and uncontrolled diabetes • Side effects include local fat atrophy and depigmentation, 1:10000 risk of infection • Only to be administered by a trained clinician
Methylprednisolone (500–1000 mg) given as pulse therapy	Intravenously	• Hospital administered • Can be effective for a severe disease flare or poorly controlled disease • Side effects include anaphylaxis, hyper-/hypotension, cardiac arrhythmias and bronchospasm

Mild side effects of steroids include:

- Flushing
- Palpitations
- Increased appetite
- Metallic taste
- Hyperactivity
- Tiredness
- Blurred vision
- Wakefulness

These side effects will settle with dose reduction and cessation of the drug.

More serious side effects can occur with higher doses and with long-term use of steroids, such as:

- Osteoporosis
- Thinning skin
- Diabetes
- Hypertension
- Muscle wasting
- Cushing's syndrome
- Adrenal suppression
- Increased infection risk
- Weight gain
- Disruption of lipid and carbohydrate metabolism
- Glaucoma and cataract

Therefore, although they can be very effective in reducing inflammation and relieving the pain of arthritis, prolonged use of steroids is not recommended (NICE 2009) due to the risk of possible long-term side effects, which outweigh the benefits. Clinical guidelines recommend that steroids should be tapered down, as 'rapidly as clinically feasible' until, ideally, their full withdrawal (Smolen et al. 2017b).

Steroids can mask the effect of infections and if used for longer than 4 weeks or in higher doses (>10 mg daily) it is likely that the immune system will be suppressed (immunosuppression). For this reason people needing to take steroids in this way are recommended to have the pneumococcal and annual flu vaccinations.

Synthetic steroids act to suppress the natural production of naturally occurring (endogenous) steroid by the adrenal cortex, particularly when used in higher doses and for more than 3 weeks. For this reason, slow dose reduction is recommended in order to allow the adrenal cortex to gradually start producing endogenous steroid again. If abruptly stopped, serious and potentially fatal adrenal crisis can occur.

Particular caution is needed in people with renal and liver impairment as the plasma concentration of corticosteroid may be increased. In addition, steroids, even at low doses, are the main cause of drug-induced osteoporosis (Briot and Roux 2015). Anyone starting steroids should have their bone density assessed and are advised to take calcium and vitamin D supplements. Additionally, for people over 65 years in whom steroid treatment is planned for more than 3 months, concomitant bisphosphonate (described in Section 9.6) is advised at the initiation of steroid use (Clunie 2007).

Summary of Main Points

1. The aim of pharmacological management in people with inflammatory arthritis is to reduce pain and inflammation, to prevent damage to joints and to halt or slow the progression of disease, enabling the person to live a normal life where possible.
2. Analgesics, NSAIDs and DMARDs may be used in combination to treat arthritis.
3. Paracetamol and topical NSAIDs are recommended as first-line treatment for people with OA.
4. NSAIDs should be used at the lowest dose for the shortest possible time.
5. Methotrexate is the first-line treatment for inflammatory arthritis.
6. DMARD drugs should be stopped if someone develops an infection.
7. Biologic drugs can safely be used in the older person.
8. Steroids can help when a person's arthritis is flaring, but oral steroids should not be stopped abruptly.
9. Due to comorbidities and a combination of physiological factors, older people are more at risk of developing adverse effects. Consequently, lower doses of drugs, regular monitoring and supervision are recommended.

9.7   Self-Assessment

The following are ideas of how you might relate and apply to practice what you have learned from this chapter:

1. Consider what would be the most effective and safe drug treatment for an elderly person with painful knees due to their OA.
2. What advice would you give to a patient who is on oral methotrexate and has a chest infection?
3. An elderly patient with inflammatory arthritis wants to stop taking her oral steroids. What advice would you give?

References

American Geriatrics Society Panel on the Pharmacological Management of Persistent Pain in older Persons. Pharmacological management of pain in older persons. J Am Geriatr Soc. 2009;57:1331–46.

Bressolle F, Bologna C, Kinowski JM, Sany J, Combe B. Effects of moderate renal insufficiency on pharmacokinetics of methotrexate in rheumatoid arthritis patients. Ann Rheum Dis. 1998;57(2):110–3.

Briot K, Roux C. Glucocorticoid-induced osteoporosis. Rheum Musculoskelet Dis Open. 2015;1:e000014. https://doi.org/10.1136/rmdopen-2014-000014.

British National Formulary 76. Sept 2018–Mar 2019. Chapter 10/4. 2018–2019. BNF.org.

Calderia D, Costa J, Barra M, et al. How safe is acetaminophen use in patients treated with vitamin K antagonists. A systematic review and meta-analysis. Thromb Res. 2015;135(1):58–61.

Cepeda M, Camargo F, Zea C, Valencia L. Tramadol for osteoarthritis. Cochrane Database Syst Rev. 2006;(3):CD005522.

Clunie G. Update on postmenopausal osteoporosis management. Clin Med. 2007;7(1):48–52.

Criswell LA, Saag G, Sems KM, et al. Moderate-term, low dose corticosteroids for rheumatoid arthritis (Cochrane Review). In: The Cochrane library, issue 1. Chichester, UK: John Wiley & Sons Ltd; 2004.

Deighton C, Hyrich K, Ding T, Ledlingham J, et al. BSR and BHPR rheumatoid arthritis guidelines on eligibility criteria for the first biologic therapy. Rheumatology. 2010;4(6):1197–9.

Emery P, Breedveld FC, Dougados M, Kalden JR, Schiff MH, Smolen JS. Early referral recommendation for newly diagnosed rheumatoid arthritis: evidence based development of a clinical guide. Ann Rheum Dis. 2002;61(4):290–7.

Fine PG. Treatment guidelines for the pharmacological management of pain in older persons. Pain Med. 2012;13:S57–66.

Fine PG, Herr KA. Pharmacological management of persistent pain in older persons. Clin Geriatr. 2009;17(4):25–32.

Fleiscmann RM, Baumgartner SW, Tindall EA, et al. Response to etanercept (Enbrel) in elderly patients with rheumatoid arthritis: a retrospective analysis of clinical trial results. J Rheumatol. 2003;30(40):691–6.

Frank RG, Kashani JH, Parker JC, Beck NC, et al. Antidepressant analgesia in rheumatoid arthritis. J Rheumatol. 1988;15:1632–8.

Furlan A, Sandoval J, Mailis-Gagnon A, Tunks E. Opioids for chronic noncancer pain: a meta-analysis of effectiveness and side effects. Can Med Assoc J. 2006;174:1589–94.

Furukawa TA, McGuire H, Barbui C. Meta-analysis of effects and side effects of low dosage tricyclic antidepressants in depression: systematic review. BMJ. 2002;325:991. https://doi.org/10.1136/bmj.325.7371.991.

Heerdink ER, Leufkens HG, Herings RM, et al. NSAIDs associated risk in congestive heart failure in elderly patients taking diuretics. Arch Intern Med. 1998;158:1108–12.

Hinz B, Brune K. Paracetamol and cyclooxygenase inhibition: is there a cause for concern? Ann Rheum Dis. 2012;71(1):20–5.

Hirshberg B, Muszkat M, Schlesinger O, Rubinow A. Safety of low dose methotrexate in elderly patients with rheumatoid arthritis. Postgrad Med. 2002;76:787–9.

Hochberg MC, Altman RD, April KT, et al. American College of Rheumatology 2012 recommendations for the use of nonpharmacologic and pharmacologic therapies in osteoarthritis of the hand, hip, and knee. Arthritis Care Res. 2012;64:465. https://doi.org/10.1002/acr.21596.

Holroyd CR, Seth R, Bukhari M, Malaviya A, et al. The British Society for Rheumatology biologic DMARD safety guidelines in inflammatory arthritis. Rheumatology. 2019;58:e3–e42. https://doi.org/10.1093/rheumatology/key208.

Keystone EC, Taylor PC, Tanaka Y, Gaich C, et al. Patient-reported outcomes from a phase 3 study of baricitinib versus placebo or adalimumab in rheumatoid arthritis: secondary analyses from the RA-BEAM study. Ann Rheum Dis. 2017;76(11):1853–61.

van Laar M, Pergolizzi JV Jr, Mellinghoff H-U, et al. Pain treatment in arthritis-related pain: beyond NSAIDs. Open Rheumatol J. 2012;6:320–30.

Ledingham J, Gullick N, Irving K, Gorodkin R, et al. BSR and BHPR guideline for the prescription and monitoring of non-biologic disease-modifying anti-rheumatic drugs. Rheumatology. 2017;56:865–8. https://doi.org/10.1093/rheumatology/kew479.

Luqmani R, Hennell S, Estrach C, Birrell A, et al. British Society for Rheumatology and British Health professional in Rheumatology guideline for the Management of Rheumatoid arthritis (the first two years). Rheumatology. 2006;45:1167–9.

McCleane G. Pharmacological pain management in the elderly patient. Clin Interv Aging. 2007;2(4):637–43.

National Institute for Health and Care Excellence. Osteoarthritis: care and management 2014 Clinical guideline [CG177]. Published date: Feb 2014. Available from: https://www.nice.org.uk/guidance/cg177/chapter/1-Recommendations#pharmacological-management. Accessed 15 Feb 2019.

NICE. The management of rheumatoid arthritis in adults. NICE clinical guideline 79. National Institute for Health and Clinical Excellence. 2009. Available from: http://publications.nice.org.uk/rheumatoid-arthritis-cg79. Accessed 13 Mar 2014.

NICE. Adalimumab, etanercept, infliximab, certolizumab pegol, golimumab, tocilizumab and abatacept for rheumatoid arthritis not previously treated with DMARDs or after conventional DMARDS have failed. Technology appraisal guidance [TA375]. Published date: 26 Jan 2016. Available from: https://www.nice.org.uk/guidance/ta375. Accessed 15 Apr 2019.

NICE. Baricitinib for moderate to severe rheumatoid arthritis. Technology appraisal guidance [TA466]. Published date: 06 Aug 2017. 2017a. Available from: https://www.nice.org.uk/guidance/ta466/chapter/1-Recommendations. Accessed 15 Apr 2019.

NICE. Tofacitinib for moderate to severe rheumatoid arthritis. Technology appraisal [TA480]. Published date: 11 Oct 2017. 2017b. Available from: https://www.nice.org.uk/guidance/ta480/chapter/1-Recommendations. Accessed 15 Apr 2019.

Rannou F, Pelletier J-P, Martel-Pelletier J. Efficacy and safety of topical NSAIDs in the management of osteoarthritis: evidence from real-life setting trials and surveys. Semin Arthritis Rheum. 2016;45:S18–21.

Robinson WH, Mao R. Biomarkers to guide clinical therapeutics in rheumatology? Curr Opin Rheumatol. 2016;28(2):168–75.

Schneeweiss S, Setoguchi S, Weinblatt ME, et al. Anti-tumour necrosis factor α therapy and the risk of serious bacterial infections in the elderly patients with rheumatoid arthritis. Arthritis Rheum. 2007;56(6):1754.

Scott DL. Advances in the medical management of rheumatoid arthritis. Hosp Med. 2002;63(5):294–7.

Simon L, Lipman SL, et al. Guidelines for the management of pain in osteoarthritis, rheumatoid arthritis and juvenile chronic arthritis. 2nd ed. Glenview, IL: American Pain Society; 2002.

Singh JA, Cameron C, Noorbaloochi S, et al. Risk of serious infection in biological treatments in patients with rheumatoid arthritis: a systematic review and meta-analysis. Lancet. 2015;386:258–65.

Smolen JS, et al. A treating rheumatoid arthritis to target: 2014 update of the recommendations of an international task force. Ann Rheum Dis. 2016;75:3–15.

Smolen JS, Landewé R, Bijlsma J, et al. EULAR recommendations for the management of rheumatoid arthritis with synthetic and biological disease-modifying antirheumatic drugs: 2016 update. Ann Rheum Dis. 2017a;76:960–77. https://doi.org/10.1136/annrheumdis-2016-210715.

Smolen JS, et al. EULAR recommendations for the management of rheumatoid arthritis with synthetic and biological disease-modifying antirheumatic drugs: 2016 update. Ann Rheum Dis. 2017b;76:960–77.

Stannard C. Opioids in the UK, whats the problem? BMJ. 2013;347:f5108.

Stannard C, Booth S. Chapter 6: Pain. In: Churchill's pocket books. 2nd ed. London: Elsevier Churchill Livingstone; 2004. p. 83–101.

Veena K, Ranganath MD, Daniel E, Furst MD. Disease-modifying antirheumatic drug use in the elderly rheumatoid arthritis patient. Rheum Dis Clin North Am. 2006;33(1):197–217.

WHO. WHO's pain ladder. Geneva, Switzerland: World Health Organization; 1986. [updated 2011]. Available from: http://www.who.int/cancer/palliative/painladder/en/. Accessed 15 Feb 2019.

Wilkieson CA, Madhok R, Hunter JA, Capell HA. Toleration, side-effects and efficacy of sulfasalazine in rheumatoid arthritis patients of different ages. Int J Med. 1993;86(8):501–5. https://doi.org/10.1093/qjmed/86.8.501.

Further Reading

Access the European League Against Rheumatism (EULAR) guidelines on the management of rheumatoid arthritis (rheumnow.com/content/2016-eular-guidelines-ra-management). Evaluate how the recommended use of DMARDs compares to practice in your local rheumatology department.

Read the National Institute for Health and Care Excellence Multimorbidity and polypharmacy. Key Therapeutic topic, Jan 2017. Updated Mar 2019 at https://www.nice.org.uk/advice/ktt18/chapter/evidence-context.

Read rheumatoid arthritis: appropriate treatment in the older person at https://onlinelibrary.wiley.com/doi/pdf/10/1002/psb.55.

Optimising Function

10

Kay Stevenson, Greg Bicker, Ben Jeeves,
and Hannah Elliott

10.1 Learning Outcomes

By the end of the chapter, the nurse will be able to:

- Describe the importance of remaining active and undertaking exercise
- Identify how to exercise and increase activity safely
- Describe how to promote activity in older people recovering from injury/surgery
- Recognise the role of other health professionals and services available to patients to optimise function

10.2 Introduction

As the number of older adults continues to increase worldwide, optimising function and encouraging physical activity is an important priority for all health professionals. Currently on average, adults over 65 years spend 10 hours or more each day sitting or lying down, making them the most sedentary age group (NHS

10

K. Stevenson (✉)
Haywood Hospital, Midlands Partnership NHS Foundation Trust, Keele University, Newcastle, Staffordshire, UK

The Impact Accelerator Unit, School of Primary, Community and Social Care, Keele University, Newcastle, Staffordshire, UK
e-mail: Kay.stevenson@mpft.nhs.uk

G. Bicker · B. Jeeves · H. Elliott
Haywood Hospital, Midlands Partnership NHS Foundation Trust, Keele University, Newcastle, Staffordshire, UK

© Springer Nature Switzerland AG 2020
S. Ryan (ed.), *Nursing Older People with Arthritis and other Rheumatological Conditions*, Perspectives in Nursing Management and Care for Older Adults, https://doi.org/10.1007/978-3-030-18012-6_10

Website 2019a). Globally older people are living with multi-morbidity; four out of five people with osteoarthritis have at least one other long-term condition such as hypertension (Musculoskeletal Conditions and Co-morbidities Arthritis Research UK 2019). Amongst people over 45 years of age who report living with major long-term conditions, more than three out of ten find it hard to live independently or well.

Musculoskeletal conditions, including osteoarthritis, affect over ten million people in the United Kingdom (UK) alone (Musculoskeletal Conditions and Co-morbidities Arthritis Research UK 2019). These conditions can cause pain, stiffness, loss of mobility, loss of dexterity and depression and are closely associated with other morbidities. Multi-morbidity is when a person has two or more long-term chronic conditions. Women often have higher rates of multi-morbidity than men (Smith 2012). Multi-morbidity reduces quality of life, leads to poorer health outcomes and increases mortality. People with multi-morbidity are frequent users of health systems, accounting for a high proportion of general practice consultations and hospital admissions in the UK. The high level of need for health care also has an impact on the patient themselves, having to attend appointments, collecting and taking regular medications and following exercise programmes.

Physical function and functional status is an important predictor of health outcomes in the older person particularly hospitalisation, surgical outcomes and mortality (Buford et al. 2014). Functional status is measured by the ability of people to perform basic activities of daily living consisting of care tasks including feeding, bathing, dressing, using the toilet, personal hygiene, transferring from bed to chair and walking. More advanced activities could include hobbies and leisure activities. There are validated screening tools available which can highlight risk factors and causes for decreasing physical function. The electronic frailty index (eFI) (NHS Website 2019b) and the timed get up and go test are two measures that are readily used (Get-Up-and-Go 2010).

The Centers for Disease Control and Prevention (CDC) programme in America (USA) has identified nine functional limitations that people with multi-morbidity in arthritis report as being very difficult or unable to do (Centres for Disease Control and Preventions Arthritis Programme 2016). These are grasping small objects, sitting for more than 2 hours, climbing a flight of stairs, walking a quarter of a mile, reaching above the head, lifting or carrying 10 pounds, pushing a heavy object and standing for greater than 2 hours. In 2010–2012 more than 43% of US citizens with arthritis could not do these activities (Centers for Disease Control and Prevention (CDC) 2013).

Functional decline in itself is not a condition but it can have a negative impact on both acute and chronic medical conditions. People who remain active over the age of 65 years have lower risk of heart disease, stroke, type 2 diabetes, some cancers, depression and dementia (NHS Website 2019a). Regular exercise can also reduce the risk of falls (NHS Website 2019a). Physical activity is one of the only interventions consistently demonstrated to prevent functional decline amongst older people (Pahor et al. 2006).

Fig. 10.1 Older people engaging in exercise

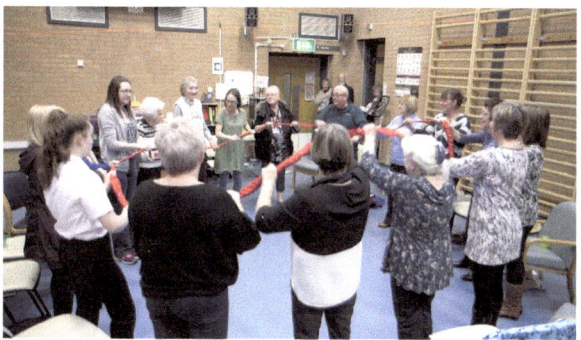

10.3   The Case for Exercise

The purpose of exercise is to maximise quality of life by reducing pain and stiffness, limiting progression of joint damage and enabling function (Zhnag 2008). Physical activity in the forms of general exercise should include both aerobic activity such as walking (see Fig. 10.1), swimming or cycling and muscle strengthening exercises such as resistance band or weights, which have been shown to reduce overall pain (Musculoskeletal Conditions and Co-morbidities Arthritis Research UK 2019).

If a person is having difficulty performing everyday activities, then a referral to occupational therapy can be a useful adjunct to promote personal independence and maintain function. For example if a person is having difficulty remaining active, for example in the garden, then an occupational therapist (OT) can look at the specific task causing a problem. Options can then be discussed for either tackling the activity in a different way (using raised beds to plant seeds) or adapting implements (padding the handles of tools to reduce pressure on the joint). Alternatively, if the older person is finding it difficult to remain active with the grandchildren, the OT can discuss planning and pacing activities to manage reduced energy levels.

Exercise can also play a significant role in mental wellbeing; 36% of older patients with multi-morbidity suffer with mental health issues. Mental wellbeing ensures that the person feels good about themselves and will affect what activities they engage in (see Chapter 8). Physical activity can help with mild depression and anxiety and can enhance self-esteem and self-control (NHS Website 2019c). The emphasis is on self-management to enable a person to maximise their potential to live a full and active life.

10.4   How to Exercise and Increase Activity Safely

Exercise broadly encompasses physical activity. There is a plethora of evidence demonstrating the association between lack of physical activity and mortality. The importance of maintaining physical activity as we age, and importantly in the context of managing health-related issues, must not be ignored. Ageing is associated with loss of muscle mass, termed age-related sarcopenia, which can have wide-reaching health implications. Such is its importance it is now recognised as a muscle disease (Cruz-Jentoft et al. 2019). Further sarcopenia increases falls risk and subsequent fractures and is associated with loss of cognitive function, cardiac and respiratory disease, lower quality of life and death. This can have wide-ranging and significant cost implications for health-care providers. Therefore, understanding, recognising and treating the effects of insufficient activity levels in patients is fundamental in the holistic health care of the older adult.

There is debate as to what constitutes the 'best' form of exercise. The perfect exercise modality does not exist, but it should be informed by patient preference and the desired outcome. For example, if improving strength is the specified goal, the focus should be towards a resistance programme, whereas endurance exercise would primarily involve lower intensity exercise over a prolonged period of time, for example, increasing the distance walked each day. An exercise programme can encompass a number of exercise modalities to achieve an improvement in physical ability by way of improving muscular strength, endurance and proprioception.

Current UK guidelines outlined by the Department of Health and Social Care (Department of Health and Social Care 2011) on physical activity for the older adult (64 years+) are shown in Fig. 10.2 as an example:

Health-care clinicians often focus exclusively on the outcome of exercise (improved strength, aerobic capacity or balance), whereas the purpose of exercise should be towards lifestyle changes, and what an individual enjoys, rather than exercise being viewed as an 'intervention'. With enjoyment comes adherence and sustained effects (see Fig. 10.3).

Physical functional limitations are a common clinical problem, associated with anxiety and depression (Backe et al. 2017). The positive effects of physical activity as a way of managing mental health, including depression, are widely documented. Joshi et al. (2016) suggest that the protective benefits to mental health were independent of exercise type and duration. However, Joshi et al. also identified that

An example exercise programme:

Aim to be active every day: Over a week, activity should add up to at least 150 minutes (2½ hours) of moderate-intensity activity in bouts of 10 minutes or more – one way to approach this is to do 30 minutes on at least 5 days a week.

Undertake physical activity to improve muscle strength on at least two days a week: This could include squats or repeated sit-to-stands, step-ups, shoulder presses, shoulder rows, wall press-ups, seated push-ups. These should be repeated in sets of 2–5 and repetitions of 5–15 depending on the appropriateness, goal and participants ability.

Older adults at risk of falls should incorporate physical activity to improve balance and co-ordination on at least 2 days a week: Challenging proprioception can include narrowing their stance whilst throwing/ catching walking/marching on an unstable surface using balance boards/ cushions/ trampette.

Fig. 10.2 Applying guidelines on physical activity in practice

Fig. 10.3 People enjoying exercise

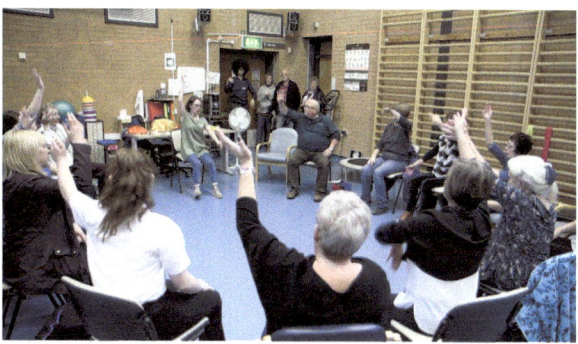

Use the word 'activity' rather than exercise.

Explore what the patient likes to do, e.g. walking, swimming, taking grandchildren to school, and walking the dog.

Try to match the activity with their daily lifestyle.

Ask the patient what they consider to be the benefits of activity.

Consider what language you use; try to use the same terminology as the patient.

Fig. 10.4 How to explain the benefits of exercise to your patient during the consultation

'high' levels of physical activity were associated with a lower risk of future depression, meaning that the benefit of physical activity may be restricted to the highest levels of and the most strenuous types of activity, suggesting a dose-dependent relationship. Therefore, achieving sufficient exercise intensity may be challenging in those with physical limitations, explaining a lack of benefit noted by patients. It is important that the clinician explains the benefits of exercise in a way that has meaning and relevance for the patient (see Fig. 10.4).

When considering the choice of exercise, a holistic approach is paramount. Consideration of the patients starting baseline fitness, co-morbidities and safety of exercise participation is required. If uncertainty exists around the safety of a patient engaging in exercise participation, consider referring to a specialist, for example, a physiotherapist, or cardiac or respiratory rehabilitation services if applicable.

It is important to consider the reasons for exercising, from the health-care practitioners' perspective, the patient's own goals and the patient's potential. Currently guidelines for physical activity for adults 65 years and older focus on the requirements of older people with no health conditions that limit their applicability (NHS Website 2019d). The guidelines do however recommend both endurance and strengthening type of exercises.

Balance exercises also play an important role in helping patients in their physical health. The reasons for reduced balance may be multi-factorial, but proprioceptive exercises (or balance exercises) may help to improve a person's balance and reduce falls risk, when part of a varied and progressive exercise regime.

10.5   Promoting Activity in Older People Recovering from Injury/Surgery or Requiring Surgery

Exercising following injury or surgery can feel intimidating to both patients and health-care professionals; subsequently seeking advice and guidance from an appropriate health professional, such as a physiotherapist, can make this process more accessible and effective.

When preparing for a surgical procedure, it is advisable for the patient to maintain mobility and strength to improve recovery post-operatively. This can be challenging due to discomfort and limitations. Many hospitals run pre-operative classes or educational programmes for patients undergoing total hip replacements (THRs) or total knee replacements (TKRs). These programmes can advise on the physical, mental and practical preparation required for the forthcoming procedure. Some services have provision for assessment or preparation of the home environment, to assist with a quicker and safer return to home post-operatively. Considerations when preparing a patient for surgery are highlighted in Fig. 10.5.

Surgical recovery times and clinical outcomes can be improved with a proactive approach to rehabilitation; this is particularly apparent in large joint replacements such as a TKR or THR. Early mobilisation or day-of-surgery mobilisation can decrease hospital length of stay and increase function; this tends to be encompassed in an enhanced recovery protocol. These protocols generally consist of a mixture of the following: pre-operation education groups, anaesthetic type and local anaesthetic infiltration, analgesic and antiemetic prophylaxis, autologous blood transfusion, catheter use and day 0 mobilisation. Together these approaches have proved highly successful in reducing hospital length of stay with high patient satisfaction in patients undergoing THR and TKR (Gwynne-Jones et al. 2017). It is difficult to delineate the benefits of individual aspects of an enhanced recovery programme, but one area that requires direct patient engagement and allows an increased perception of self-control from a patient perspective is early mobilisation and activity. Commonly nursing staff and therapists work together to encourage exercises and mobility post-operatively.

Provide information about the procedure and any specific limitations post-operatively. e.g. mobility or walking aid use following THR and TKR.

Provide information about recovery both in hospital and in the community: This may involve discussions regarding pain management and medication use.

Discuss social support network: This may involve washing and dressing support, food preparation and household duties, Stocking up on essentials and making everyday items easily accessible, e.g. crockery, cutlery and cooking utensils on the worktop rather than an inaccessible cupboard.

Equipment can be provided preoperatively to facilitate discharge post-operatively: This allows time for patients to try the equipment, e.g. raised toilet seat.

Advice on exercise pre-operatively to optimise function and improve recovery.

If no support is available, planning for care packages can be initiated.

Fig. 10.5 Considerations when preparing for surgery

Once the surgical procedure is carried out, there will be regular orthopaedic review as well as physiotherapy input; this will involve, at a minimum, mobility progression and exercise. Precautions following major joint replacements are detailed in Fig. 10.6. An occupational therapist may be involved in preparing patients for discharge home, ensuring that personal independence is optimised and the home environment is appropriate and safe. It may be appropriate for care packages to be initiated to support discharge, but ideally independence or familial support would be encouraged.

Other surgical procedures will have locally agreed protocols. Often a therapist will see patients post-operatively and explain the rehabilitation process, which can involve a home-based exercise programme or face-to-face therapy treatment sessions.

Post-operative protocols for rotator cuff repairs commonly, but not always, involve using a sling for a period of immobilisation, with gentle assisted exercises prescribed initially. Exercises are generally progressed according to tissue healing times and pain limitations. As with large joint replacements, the effect on independence and function of any surgical procedure should be considered prior to a patient returning home from hospital. The ability of the patient to perform daily activities needs to be considered; for patients undergoing upper limb surgery, use of the dominant hand, including washing, dressing and meal preparation, needs to be assessed.

The main limiting factors in post-operative rehabilitation tend to be pain and apprehension. Reassuring patients can be effective along with utilisation of appropriate analgesia to assist in a timely recovery.

Sudden changes in function or pain or a history of post-operative trauma can all be cause for concern and may require urgent medical or surgical review. Potential post-operative complications are shown in Fig. 10.7.

No driving for 6 weeks.

Follow wound care advice regarding washing (dependent on local protocol).

THR: (please refer to local protocols) 6-week restriction on hip flexion past 90 degrees, no crossing legs and no twisting in standing, lying or sitting. Patient must sleep on their back to avoid dislocation of the joint.

TKR: do not sleep or rest with a pillow under the knee as this will make full straightening of the knee difficult.

Fig. 10.6 Precautions post-THR and post-TKR

Excessive redness.
Heat.
Swelling.
Increasing pain.
Patient generally feeling unwell.
The patients temperature may be elevated if an infection is present.

Fig. 10.7 Potential post-operative complications

10.6   The Role of the Multi-Disciplinary Team

Physiotherapists are trained in prescribing exercise to promote recovery at appropriate time points. This is useful in recovering from surgery or an injury and also in symptom management in conditions such as rheumatoid arthritis. Generally, a graded return to activity and maintenance of this activity level is recommended. Use of goal setting can be beneficial, whether this takes the form of a specific range of movement, distance walked or weight lifted. These goals can be a useful target that allow for progression in a timely manner. Often formal outcome measures are utilised by physiotherapists to objectify symptoms and progress. These can range simply from 0–10 numerical rating of pain to more specific joint-related scores or measure for function including the Oswestry Disability Index Questionnaire (Fairbank and Pynsent 2000) or the MSKHQ (Hill et al. 2016). These measures can also be used as a motivational tracking tool and a guide for patient progression.

In the UK patients have the option to be seen by a physiotherapist as a first point of contact instead of a GP (Chartered Society of Physiotherapy 2018). Physiotherapists are highly trained to assess and manage patients with musculoskeletal disease, but in this capacity they also have the ability to refer into specialised services such as clinical assessment and treatment centres (CATS) that have additional knowledge and diagnostic services available (Roddy et al. 2010).

Self-referral to physiotherapy has been available in Scotland since a large study in 2007 demonstrated it had a positive effect on patient outcomes (Holdsworth et al. 2007). A subsequent pilot study in the UK which explored the feasibility of direct access to physiotherapy suggested there was good uptake and no evidence that it led to increased waiting times in physiotherapy and it was safe (Bishop et al. 2017).

Getting the right care for older patients with arthritis is crucial. A stratified care approach for patients with low back pain improves patient outcome and was cost effective (Hill et al. 2011). Stratified care means assessing the level of clinical need and matching treatment to that need. For those with back pain, this means assessing patient levels of risk of ongoing disability and matching the care specifically to that risk, whilst group-based rehabilitation programme for patients with chronic knee pain improved physical function and were cost effective (Hurley et al. 2012).

To optimise function in older people who have a rheumatological condition, nurses may need to seek the support of other professionals who have special expertise in this area. These include podiatrists, occupational therapists, rheumatologists, orthopaedic surgeons and pain specialists. It is important to understand the key contributions of each individual professional and how to access their services as this may vary depending on geographical location. For the majority of time, older people manage and seek assistance and support from friends and family. However, there may be occasions when pain levels increase or function starts to deteriorate, and it is important that during these times additional help is sought (also see Chapter 12).

10.7   Factors that Can Impact on Function

Function may be affected by:

- Worsening pain (see Chapter 7)
- Joint swelling
- Joint stiffness
- Disturbed sleep
- Fatigue (see Chapter 6)
- Decreasing ability to walk
- Difficulties with everyday tasks, including climbing stairs, problems with dressing or washing independently and difficulty managing tasks around the home

10.8   The Impact of Mood on Function

There is a clear link between rheumatological/MSK problems and mental health (Arthritis Research UK 2017). Four out of five people with osteoarthritis have at least one other long-term condition including depression (State of Musculoskeletal Health Arthritis 2019). A low mood state is likely to impact on patients trying to remain active, and consequently the nurse will need to be aware of the older person's psychological status. In a large musculoskeletal interface service in the UK, a third of the patients presenting to the service had anxiety and depression (Roddy et al. 2010), and 75% of patients had experienced pain for over 1 year. Clinical audits of the same population showed high levels of inactivity. Whilst 80% of patients receiving a total knee replacement do very well, 20% of patients at 12 months still have ongoing pain. A poor outcome is more prevalent in people with anxiety and depression and multi-site pain (Santaguida et al. 2008; Gandi et al. 2010). See Chapter 8.

10.9   The Role of Voluntary Services

Voluntary sector organisations can assist older patients to manage their condition and optimise their function. Recognised charities within the UK such as National Ankylosing Spondylitis Society (NASS), Arthritis Care and the National Rheumatoid Arthritis Society (NRAS) and Arthritis and Musculoskeletal Alliance (ARMA) have self-help groups that promote engagement, participation and activity. Locally, there may be rambling or walking groups, walking football/netball or Tai Chi (Wang et al. 2018), all of which promote physical activity in the older person and a positive change in health.

10.10 Conclusion

All health-care professionals caring for patients with a rheumatological/MSK condition have the opportunity to promote activity and a healthy lifestyle. Through their interactions, they can see how the physical, social and emotional consequence of living with a long-term condition may be impacting on function. By having knowledge of the health and voluntary sector services available, older people can be supported to receive the care required to optimise their function.

Summary of the Main Points
1. There is an increasing ageing population who will need to remain fit and active.
2. Physical function is an important predictor of health outcome.
3. Exercise can reduce pain and stiffness and improve wellbeing.
4. Physiotherapists and occupational therapists can assist patients in gaining confidence to undertake activity and exercise.
5. Promote balance (proprioception), strengthening and endurance exercises when prescribing activity.
6. Exercising before and after surgery can improve outcome and assist recovery.
7. Voluntary services may assist patients in self-management.

10.11 Self-Assessment

Assessing your own learning and performance needs regarding optimising function in the older person. Having read the chapter and undertaken further study, the following are some ideas as to how to relate what you have learnt to your practice:

1. How would you explain the benefits of remaining active to a patient?
2. What activities would you recommend to an older patient with knee osteoarthritis to optimise their function?
3. What activity advice would you give to a patient following a total hip replacement?
4. Discuss with a colleague the role of the physiotherapist in supporting an older person to remain active.

References

Arthritis Research UK. Musculoskeletal conditions and multimorbidity. 2017.
Backe IF, Patil GG, Nes RB, Clench-Aas J. The relationship between physical functional limitations, and psychological distress: considering a possible mediating role of pain, social support and sense of mastery. SSM Popul Health. 2017;4:153–63. Published 22 Dec 2017. https://doi.org/10.1016/j.ssmph.2017.12.005.

Bishop A, Ogollah R, Jowett S, Kigozi J, Tooth S, Protheroe J, et al. STEMS pilot trial: a pilot cluster randomised trial to investigate the addition of patient direct access to physiotherapy two usual GP LED primary care for adults with musculoskeletal pain. BMJ Open. 2017;7(3):e012987.

Buford TW, Anton SD, Clark DJ, Higgins TJ, Cooke MB. Optimizing the benefits of exercise on physical function in older adults. PM R. 2014;6(6):528–43. https://doi.org/10.1016/j.pmrj.2013.11.009.

Centers for Disease Control and Prevention (CDC). Prevalence of doctor diagnosed arthritis and arthritis attributable activity limitation—United States, 2010–2012. MMWR Morb Mortal Wkly Rep. 2013;62(44):869–73.

Centres for Disease Control and Preventions Arthritis Programme. 2016. https://www.cdc.gov/arthritis/datastatisitcs/disabilites-limitations.htm. Last accessed 27 May 2019.

Chartered Society of Physiotherapy first contact physiotherapists in general practice—a guide for implementation in England. May 2018, v. 3. https://www.csp.org.uk/system/files/001404_fcp_guidance_england_2018.pdf. Accessed 27 May 2019.

Cruz-Jentoft AJ, Bahat G, Bauer J, Boire Y, Bruyere O, Cederholm T, Cooper C, Landi F, Rolland Y, Sayer AA, Schneider SM, Sieber CC, Topinkova E, Vandewoude M, Visser M, Zamboni M, Writing Group for the European Working Group on Sarcopenia in Older People 2 (EWGSOP2), and the Extended Group for EWGSOP2. Sarcopenia: revised European consensus on definition and diagnosis. Age Ageing. 2019;48:16–31.

Department of Health and Social Care. 2011. UK physical activity guidelines. https://www.gov.uk/government/publications/uk-physical-activity-guidelines. Accessed May 2019.

Fairbank JC, Pynsent PB. The Oswestry Disability Index. Spine. 2000;25(22):2940–52; discussion 52.

Gandi R, Dhotar H, Razak F, Tso P, Davey R, Mahomed NL. Predicting the longer term outcomes of total knee arthroplasty. Knee. 2010;17:15–8. National Joint Registry England and Wales 8th annual report.

Get-Up-and-Go (timed and modified), Single Limb Stance Test, Functional Reach. [3] American Geriatrics Society. AGS/BGS clinical practice guideline: prevention of falls in older persons. 2010. http://www.medcats.com/FALLS/frameset.htm. http://www.medcats.com/. Last accessed 19 Dec 2016.

Gwynne-Jones, et al. Enhanced recovery after surgery for hip and knee replacements. Orthop Nurs. 2017;36(3):203–10.

Hill JC, Whitehurst DGT, Lewis M, Bryan S, Dunn KM, Foster NE, Konstantinou K, Main CJ, Mason E, Somerville S, Sowden G, Vohora K, Hay EM. Comparison of stratified primary care management for low back pain with current best practice (STarT Back): a randomised controlled trial. Lancet. 2011;378:1560.

Hill JC, Kang S, Benedetto E, et al. Development and initial cohort validation of the Arthritis Research UK Musculoskeletal Health Questionnaire (MSK-HQ) for use across musculoskeletal care pathways. BMJ Open. 2016;6:e012331. https://doi.org/10.1136/bmjopen-2016012331.

Holdsworth, et al. What are the costs to NHS Scotland of self referral to physiotherapy? Results of a national trial. Physiotherapy. 2007;93(1):3–11.

Hurley LMV, Walsh NE, Mitchell H, Nicholas J, Patel A. Long-term outcomes and costs of an integrated rehabilitation program for chronic knee pain: a pragmatic, cluster randomized, controlled trial. Arthritis Care Res (Hoboken). 2012;64(2):238–47. https://doi.org/10.1002/acr.20642.

Joshi S, Mooney SJ, Kennedy GJ, et al. Beyond METs: types of physical activity and depression among older adults. Age Ageing. 2016;45(1):103–9. https://doi.org/10.1093/ageing/afv164.

Musculoskeletal Conditions and Co-morbidities Arthritis Research UK. 2019. https://doi.org/www.versusarthritis.org/media/14594/state-of-musculoskeletal-health-2019.pdf. Accessed 27 May 2019.

NHS Website. 2019a. https://www.nhs.uk/live-well/exercise/exercise-as-you-get-older/. Accessed 27 May 19.

NHS Website. 2019b. https://www.england.nhs.uk/ourwork/clinical-policy/older-people/frailty/efi/. Last accessed 27 May 2019.

NHS Website. 2019c. https://www.nhs.uk/conditions/stress-anxiety-depression/mental-benefits-of-exercise/. Accessed 27 May 19.

NHS Website. 2019d. https://www.nhs.uk/live-well/exercise/physical-activity-guidelines-older-adults/. Accessed 27 May 2019.

Pahor M, Blain SN, Espland M, Fielding R, Gill TM, Gurtlnick JM, Hadley EC, King AL, Meraldi C, Miller ME, Newman AB, Relcski WJ, Rmasticken S, Stodenski S. Effects of a physical activity intervention on measures of physical performance: results of the lifestyle interventions and independence, the elders pilot study. J Gerontol A Biol Sci Med Sci. 2006;61(11):1157–65.

Roddy E, Zwierska I, Dawes P, Hider SL, Jordan KP, Packham J, Stevenson K, Hay E, SAMBA Team. The Staffordshire arthritis, musculoskeletal, and back assessment (SAMBA) study: a prospective observational study of patient outcome following referral to a primary-secondary care musculoskeletal interface service. BMC Musculoskelet Disord. 2010;11:67.

Santaguida PL, Hawker GA, Hudak PL, Glazier R, Mahomed NN, Kreder HJ, Coyte PC, Wright JG. Patient characteristics affecting the prognosis of total hip and knee arthroplasty: a systematic review. Can J Surg. 2008;51(6):428–36.

Smith. Managing patients with multi morbidity: systematic review of interventions in primary care and community settings. BMJ. 2012;345:e5205.

State of Musculoskeletal Health Arthritis and other musculoskeletal conditions in numbers. 2019. https://www.versusarthritis.org/about-arthritis/healthcare-professionals/network-news/august-2019-network-news/the-state-of-musculoskeletal-health-annual-report-for-2019/. Accessed 3 Jan 2019.

Wang C, Schmid CH, Fielding RA, Harvey WF, Reid KF, Price LL, et al. Effect of tai chi versus aerobic exercise for fibromyalgia: comparative effectiveness randomized controlled trial. BMJ. 2018;360:k851.

Zhnag. OARSI recommendations for the management of hip and knee osteoarthritis: OARSI evidence based, expert consensus guidelines. Osteoarthritis Cartilage. 2008;16(2):137–62.

Further Reading

Evans M. 23.5 hour Dr Mike Evans – You Tube. https://www.youtube.com/watch?v=aUaInS6HIGo.

Foster NE, Healey EL, Nicholls E, Holden MA, Tooth S, Hay EM. Clinical effectiveness of enhanced exercise therapy for adults with knee osteoarthritis. 3 year follow-up a randomised controlled trial (the beep trial). Osteoarthr Cartil. 2019;27:S488–9.

Quicke JG, Foster NE, Thomas MJ, Holden MA. Is long-term physical activity safe for older adults with knee pain?: a systematic review. Osteoarthr Cartil. 2015;23(9):1445–56.

Teo PL, Hinman RS, Egerton T, Dziedzic KS, Bennell KL. Identifying and prioritizing clinical guideline recommendations most relevant to physical therapy practice for hip and/or knee osteoarthritis. J Orthop Sports Phys Ther. 2019;49(7):501–12.

The Foot

11

Anita Williams

11.1 Learning Outcomes

At the end of this chapter, the nurse will be able to:

1. Describe how rheumatic diseases and aging can affect the feet.
2. Identify the foot problems associated with rheumatic diseases and aging.
3. Identify the problems/serious foot health complications associated with some rheumatic diseases that require urgent referral to the appropriate specialist.
4. Identify common foot problems, such as skin and nail pathologies, and structural/functional problems that need referring for specialist foot care/intervention.
5. Provide basic foot care advice.

11.2 Introduction

Feet are complex structures made up of 26 bones (Fig. 11.1) and 33 joints with an intricate arrangement of interlacing muscles, tendons and ligaments. The normal function of these structures is to allow feet to move and adapt freely to the surface being walked upon and the activities being undertaken. Feet are responsible for transferring our body weight from one foot to the other during weight-bearing activities such as walking or running. Providing shock absorption as feet strike the ground with each step and providing a 'stable' platform from which weight-bearing activities can be carried out.

A. Williams (✉)
School of Health and Society, University of Salford, Salford, UK
e-mail: A.E.Williams1@salford.ac.uk

© Springer Nature Switzerland AG 2020
S. Ryan (ed.), *Nursing Older People with Arthritis and other Rheumatological Conditions*, Perspectives in Nursing Management and Care for Older Adults,
https://doi.org/10.1007/978-3-030-18012-6_11

Fig. 11.1 The bones of the feet (1. calcaneum; 2. talus; 3. navicular; 4–6 cuneiforms; 7 cuboid; 8–12 metatarsals; 13–17 and unlabelled bones phalanges)

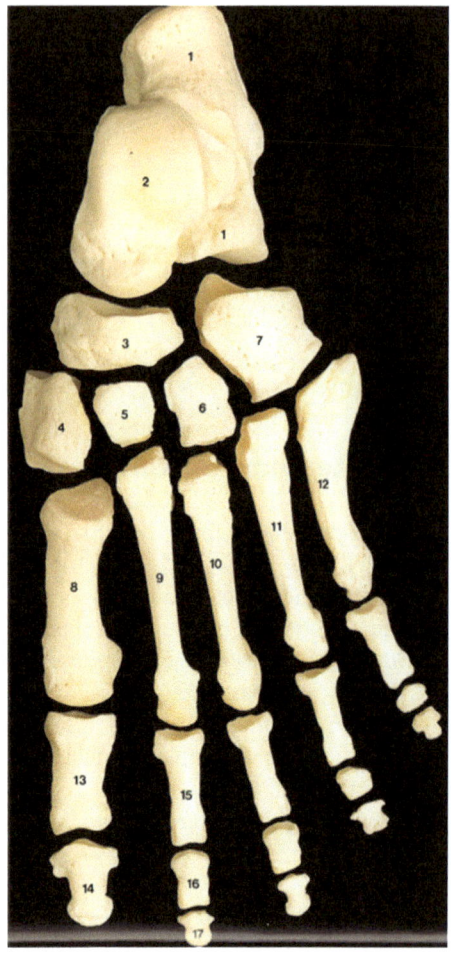

However, there are many extrinsic and intrinsic factors that affect normal function of the feet. Extrinsic factors include incorrect footwear (Menz and Morris 2005), excessive periods of activity such as in certain occupations and the environment (including temperature and terrain). Intrinsic factors include conditions which can be inherited or acquired. Examples of acquired conditions are rheumatic diseases such as rheumatoid arthritis, systemic lupus erythematosus and gout to name a few. These rheumatic diseases affect the feet in various ways, but commonly inflammation and joint involvement leads to changes in foot structure, reduction in joint mobility and foot pain which, in turn, lead to limited activity and disability. Hence, foot problems and pain have a significant impact on quality of life (Wickman et al. 2004; McElhone et al. 2010). These are further compounded by the effects of aging where the anatomical structures become weaker and the fibro fatty pad that protects the underside of the forefoot becomes thinner with subsequent pain. Foot pain is associated with decreased ability to perform activities of daily living and problems with balance and falls in both the elderly (Menz et al. 2018) and those with rheumatic diseases (Brenton-Rule et al. 2016).

Despite foot problems being common, they are under-reported by both patients and the rheumatology team (Blake et al. 2013; Williams and Graham 2012), and this reduces the potential for early diagnosis of rheumatic diseases (Emery et al. 2002) and the commencement of effective foot health interventions. Hence, it is vital that all health professionals can identify foot problems, provide advice and refer appropriately.

Rheumatoid arthritis and systemic lupus erythematosus will be used as two examples of the rheumatic diseases that manifest in the feet from the early stages of the disease. Indeed, the feet are often the first place that symptoms present and, in that respect, can aid diagnosis. The effects of aging compound the problems that are associated with these rheumatic diseases. Further, common foot problems such as skin and nail infections have more serious consequences than the general population due to the autoimmune nature of some of these diseases. Therefore, it is vital that nurses can identify symptoms in the foot that may indicate a possible rheumatic disease. As well as identifying problems in those patient with diagnosed rheumatic disease that need referring for professional foot care and to be able to provide advice for good foot health and self-care.

11.3 Rheumatoid Arthritis and the Feet

Up to 90% of people with rheumatoid arthritis will report associated foot problems (Grondal et al. 2008). Although any synovial joint may be affected, RA is a condition that can affect the feet (Turner et al. 2006). The foot is often the first area of the body to be systematically afflicted by RA, and at diagnosis, 16% of patients may have foot joint involvement progressing to 90% as the disease duration progresses (Grondal et al. 2008). Shi et al. (2000) states that virtually 100% of patients report foot problems within 10 years of disease onset with the degree of disability progressing early with disease duration of less than 2 years (Turner et al. 2006). The presence of foot complaints, both in early and in the chronic stage of RA, has been shown to be extremely detrimental to patients' daily lives and activities, especially ambulation (Wickman et al. 2004).

The basic pathological changes in the rheumatoid foot result from synovitis and bursitis (Hooper et al. 2012) and tenosynovitis (Barn et al. 2013), coupled with mechanical stress (Turner and Woodburn 2008). These structural and functional changes often affect gait and mobility (Turner et al. 2006). Specifically, the most common foot deformities in RA patients are hallux valgus (bunions), retraction of the lesser toes and splaying of the forefoot (Göksel Karatepe et al. 2010) (Fig. 11.2). Synovitis of the metatarsophalangeal joints can have a destructive impact on the quality and structure of the joints (Siddle et al. 2012a; Riente et al. 2006), and the surrounding soft tissues and bursitis affect the inter metatarsal bursae (Hooper et al. 2012) and contribute to forefoot deformity, pain and stiffness (Table 11.1). Tenosynovitis and midfoot synovitis lead to the development of pes plano valgus

Fig. 11.2 Early changes in the feet caused by rheumatoid arthritis, retraction of the toes, hallux abducto valgus (bunions), prominence of the metatarsophalangeal joints and separation of the toes (daylight sign)

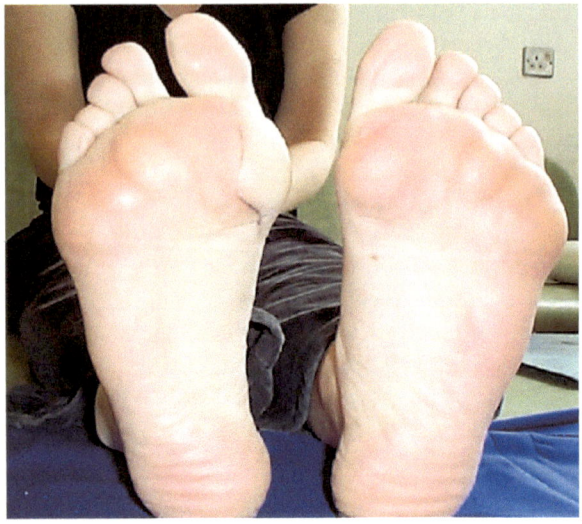

Table 11.1 Trinity of signs as a screening tool for potential early RA (Emery et al. 2002)

1. Three or more swollen joints
2. Pain on lateral compression of metatarsophalangeal joints (positive squeeze test across the forefoot)
3. Morning stiffness of 30+ mins duration

deformity (Barn et al. 2013). These foot problems result in disability in weight-bearing activities and abnormal gait patterns (Turner et al. 2008). The feet can remain symptomatic even when the disease is in remission, and despite current early medical intervention and targeted therapy (Emery et al. 2002), foot problems are still evident. Indeed there is a window of opportunity for early targeted therapy of RA-related structural foot problems (Woodburn et al. 2010), and hence referral for foot health interventions such as foot orthoses is vital in the early stages.

Persistent synovitis of the forefoot is associated with periarticular erosion, sub-luxation and dislocation of the MTP joints which in term exposes the metatarsal heads to increase pressure during gait (van der Leeden et al. 2010). In response to increased focal stresses, the skin thickens initially as a normal physiological response to chronic excessive pressure or friction of the skin. Eventually, however, this thickening of the skin called callus causes pain and contributes to impairment of gait and related functional and health status in people with RA. Shape changes in the front of the foot and the toes can also create pressure sites that develop callus and also corns (hard localised areas of skin with a harder central core or nucleus).

Some people with RA can experience decreased blood supply to feet and legs associated with atherosclerosis (Siddle et al. 2012b). Other disorders such as Raynaud's phenomena affect the small blood vessels in the skin of the hands and feet, and they 'shut down' in response to changes in temperature leading to the following colour changes: toes/fingers go white, then blue and then red. In rare cases people with RA can develop vasculitis which is inflammation of the blood vessels (McEntegart et al. 2001). This is usually associated with long-term disease, and the risks of it occurring are increased by smoking. These problems will affect tissue viability (skin thinning) and places the foot at more risk of ulceration, tissue necrosis (black areas on the toes) and even loss of toes. Some people may also experience peripheral neuropathy which is loss of protective sensation, and this can also contribute to foot ulceration (Siddle et al. 2012b).

As the foot shape alters and there is a decrease in tissue viability (associated with vascular changes and/or side effects of medication and loss of protective sensation), this can leave the feet vulnerable to ulceration (Firth et al. 2008). Further to this, bacterial and fungal skin infections and nail pathologies are more prevalent in this patient group adding to the serious risk of ulceration and systemic infection. The risk of opportunistic infections is increased if the patient's medical management is with immunosuppressive drugs (Dixon et al. 2006). Some medications used to treat RA such as steroids, DMARDS (such as methotrexate, sulfasalazine, leflunomide, azathioprine, penicillamine and injectable gold) and the biologic drugs (such as etanercept, abatacept, infliximab, adalimumab, golimumab, certolizumab, tocilizumab and rituximab) can also have an effect on the skin and underlying tissues, making them more vulnerable to damage and infection (see Chapter 9).

11.4 Systemic Lupus Erythematosus and the Feet

A UK-based survey (Cherry et al. 2017) of self-reported foot problems in those with systemic lupus erythematosus (SLE) demonstrated a wide range of foot problems associated with the condition. Whilst the relative prevalence of sensory loss was low, a quarter of the 182 participants reported having had a fall related to changes in foot sensation. Importantly, this patient population are already at increased fracture risk due to comorbid health needs and/or treatments, and therefore there is a potentially large detrimental consequence of falling.

There is also a high prevalence of vascular complications and symptoms, including tissue necrosis, reduced tissue viability and blue/black toes (Cherry et al. 2017). Advice and screening at each consultation is recommended to detect and treat early changes and reduce the risk of serious progressive consequences such as ulceration and loss of digits.

Foot problems that are prevalent in the general population such as corns, callus and nail thickening are also evident. In addition, fungal and viral infections can become more widespread due to the autoimmune nature of SLE and the immunosuppressive medication that can be used for its management.

Further, musculoskeletal problems are also common and can result in an inability to walk, have a high potential for reduced mobility (Williams et al. 2016) and subsequently may have far reaching impact on comorbid health complications (e.g. further compromise of vascular status or tissue viability). Commonly seen are flat feet (lowered or flattened arch), deformities in the toes and swelling at the back of the heel.

11.5   Management of Foot Problems

The management goal of the RA foot is reducing the pain in the feet, improving foot function, mobility (see Chapter 10) and quality of life using safe and cost-effective treatments, such as palliative foot care, prescribed foot orthoses and specialist footwear aimed at preventing any deterioration in the tissues and in joint alignment (Grondal et al. 2008; Woodburn and Helliwell 1997). Woodburn et al. also suggest that there is 'Window of Opportunity' (Woodburn et al. 2010) in early rheumatoid arthritis for effective podiatry intervention and this can also apply to SLE where structural foot problems may well be preventable. The focus of managing feet affected by RA and SLE is around monitoring circulation and nerve supply, maintaining foot structure and prevention of ulceration and infection (Cherry et al. 2017; Williams et al. 2016; ARMA Guidelines 2004).

Given that podiatrists are considered the experts in the management of foot and ankle problems and recognised by NICE (NICE 2009) as primary provider of foot health services for this patient group, they should be an integrated part of the MDT. This view is supported by ARMA (ARMA Guidelines 2004; ARMA 2004), which advocates the need for a dedicated and specialist podiatry service for the diagnosis, assessment and management of foot problems along with periodic review. Further, patient organisations (Versus Arthritis and the National Rheumatoid Arthritis Society, Lupus UK) also recommend that patients have access to specialist foot care. Podiatrists in the United Kingdom must be registered with the Health and Care Professions Council. The podiatrist role is to identify, diagnose and treat disorders, diseases and deformities of the feet and legs and implement appropriate and timely care. The goal of the podiatry element of rheumatology care is to reduce foot-related pain, maintain/improve foot function and therefore mobility whilst protecting skin and other tissues from damage.

Podiatrists can carry out an assessment of the feet and lower limbs including:

- Assessment of tissue viability—skin problems such as corns and callus, potential infections such as fungal infections.
- Vascular and neurological assessment.
- Assessment of the joints and soft tissue structures. This can be clinical and/or with ultrasonography.
- Assessment of gait, function and mobility (including risk of falls) together with assessment of footwear.

Treatments may include:

- Management of nail conditions such as thickened fungal nails or ingrowing toe nails.
- Treatment of callus and corns.
- Management of foot ulcers.
- Provision of specialist orthoses for the feet.

- Assessment and advice about appropriate footwear choices, footwear adaptations and accessing specialist footwear services. Some health service departments have footwear clinics, either independently or in association with an orthotist or shoe-fitter.
- Advice related to the lower limb including joint protection, management of acute and chronic inflamed joints, appropriate exercise and potential surgical options.

11.6 Patient Education Related to Foot Health

Podiatry-based research shows that identifying health education needs and provision of supportive verbal and written information can foster an effective therapeutic relationship, supporting effective foot health education (Graham et al. 2017). Patient education should aim to include:

- *Maintenance of foot hygiene*—washing and drying feet well, especially between the toes and being carried out on a daily basis.
- *Aspects of self-care* (using emollients on dry hard skin rather than removing callus with sharp instruments or using preparatory corn removal preparations).
- *Information regarding changes in foot health that should prompt further investigation*—increased pain, changes in skin colour especially if painful and any symptoms such as itchiness, burning, problems with nails such as ingrown nails, thickening and odour of the nails which may indicate fungal infection, itchiness and white skin between the toes may indicate fungal infection.
- *Advice regarding retail footwear suitability*—avoiding high-heeled court shoes for high usage (see section on footwear).
- *Access to podiatry* either health services or private providers (as long as HCPC registered) of podiatry care.

11.7 Foot Orthoses

The benefits of foot orthoses (insoles) and footwear have been recognised and recommended (NICE 2009). For the purposes of clarity foot orthoses and footwear options will be discussed separately. However, the practitioner should always consider them together in relation to footwear suitability, choice of foot orthoses and the potential mechanical effect of the footwear on not just the foot but the orthoses as well.

It is demonstrated that foot orthoses not only achieve pain reduction in the early RA foot but have a sustained effect on the foot structure and hence achieve stability of the joints of the foot and improve the patient's mobility (Woodburn et al. 2002). As foot changes have the potential to occur within 2 years of disease onset (Turner et al. 2006), it is essential that patients are referred for assessment of foot function as early as possible following diagnosis. Hard contoured foot orthoses are provided to improve the function of the foot and/or lower limb. This assumes that there is some mobility in the joints of the foot to improve function and realign the bony architecture.

Foot orthoses can minimise the pain and disability associated with RA when there is established foot deformity. Once the structural problems are established and joint mobility is reduced, management consists of reducing symptoms of pain and resultant mobility problems. Further to this, redistributing foot pressures may contribute to the prevention of tissue breakdown and ulceration over high pressure areas of the foot. Customised accommodative orthoses (total contact orthoses) are designed so that the material follows closely the contours of the underside of the foot. The purpose is to redistribute the pressures applied to the foot by standing and walking more evenly. This is particularly useful where there are areas of increased pressure, for example, under the metatarsal heads. In this instance, the pressure is shifted to areas of the foot that do not normally bear weight such as the arch area (Li et al. 2000). They are particularly used where there is limited or no joint mobility such as in the established RA foot and where tissue viability is poor. These orthoses are often made from materials that also provide a cushioning effect.

Although there is no evidence to support the use of foot orthoses in early or established structural foot problems associated with SLE, it is recognised by clinical experts that these are useful in relieving symptoms and improving function.

11.8   Footwear

The right footwear is essential to maintaining function, resting symptomatic joints and preventing or limiting structural foot problems in both RA and SLE. Where disease control with medical management is relatively good, addressing the mechanical causes of foot problems *before* changes in the feet become well developed can have significant benefits.

There are many manufacturers of high street footwear that provide a variety of styles and widths which will accommodate most feet and foot problems (see the Footwear Section on the NRAS web site: https://www.nras.org.uk/). It is difficult to recommend manufacturers and styles as all feet are different. These differences are not just in length but in the width of the forefoot, depth over the toes and the instep, arch height, flexibility of the joints and angle of the toes to name just a few of the variations. Patients need to know not to rely on shoe size alone as it is the fit of the shoe and how they feel in the shoes that is important.

Some people may have footwear prescribed especially for them by their consultant, GP or podiatrist. The shoes are usually provided by an orthotist who works in the orthotic services of NHS Trusts or privately. Each hospital or health service will have its own arrangements for footwear referral and entitlements. This footwear can be what is termed 'stock footwear' which is extra deep and wide or made to measure (bespoke) footwear made to a last specifically for their feet. Styles are often limited in comparison with retail footwear, and you may wish to discuss options with the patient and look at the styles available. Some patients find the cosmesis of this footwear to be an issue (Williams et al. 2011), so referral does need to be based on agreement and understanding of what to expect. It has been found that patients considered that it was important to receive information at the point of referral so that they can make considered choices as to whether to be referred for this footwear or not (van Netten et al. 2017). Without some knowledge of what is available, the opportunity to engage the patient in the decision making at this stage is lost and may be one of the reasons patient expectations are not met. The option of referral for a surgical opinion should be offered as an alternative to referral for footwear.

It is generally considered that the following patients could be considered for referral for specialist footwear for the following reasons:

- Failing to obtain retail footwear to fit the dimensions of the foot (including asymmetry)
- Pressure symptoms such as skin lesions/sore areas on the feet
- Increasing foot pain due to pressure from existing footwear
- Excessive footwear 'wear' indicating that patients need more stability from increased surface area of the plantar aspect of the footwear and increased rear-foot control from the heel counter
- History of foot ulceration where footwear has been a contributory factor

11.9   Management of Callus

Callus (hard skin) can occur on any part of the foot where there is excessive pressure such as overlying bursa on the plantar aspect of the foot (Fig. 11.3) and on the dorsum of the toes where the footwear may rub and cause callus and corns (Fig. 11.4).

Fig. 11.3 Superficial plantar callus (hard skin)

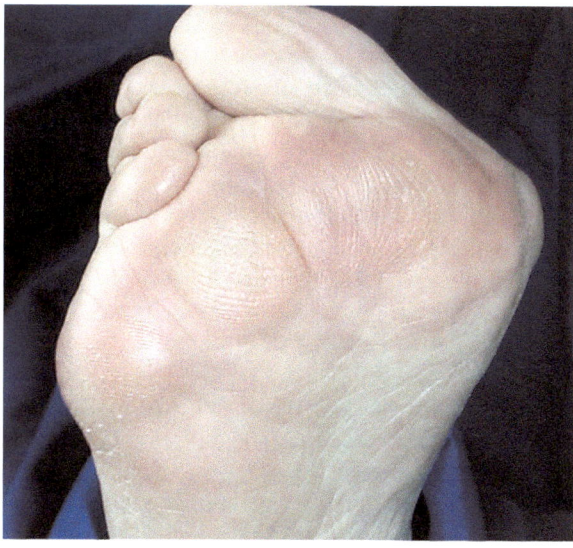

Fig. 11.4 Callus on the dorsum of the fourth toe

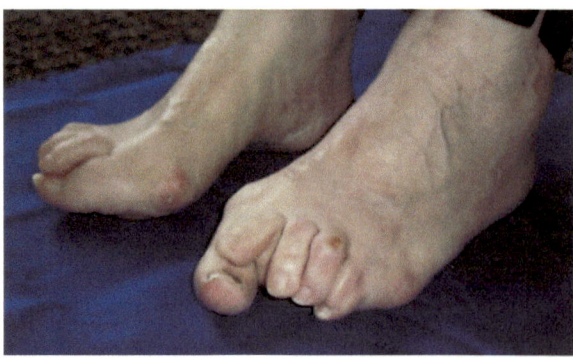

Those patients with foot deformity and/or reduced tissue viability (often associated with long-term steroid therapy, vasculitis, concurrent peripheral vascular disease) should not remove callus themselves (Siddle et al. 2013). Indeed, they should not request that podiatrists remove the callus as this may lead to ulceration. Often the pain associated with the callus is from the underlying structures as it has been shown that removal of the callus does not reduce pain compared to those who did not have the callus removed (Davys et al. 2005). However, podiatrist may remove callus if there are clinical signs of infection (such as increased pain, redness, heat and swelling) and the potential for underlying ulceration. Advice about the use of emollients for dry plantar callus should be given and patients can be advised to use a foot file on these areas at least three times a week in order to reduce the thickness gently.

11.10 Foot Ulceration

It is likely that ulcers in RA and SLE are multifactorial in origin, and these factors may contribute to the poor rates of healing. A combination of altered foot structure increasing the pressure on the feet, poor tissue viability and inappropriate footwear are the key risk factors (Firth et al. 2008; Williams et al. 2013). Foot ulceration can be recurrent; multiple sites are common and often take a long time to achieve healing which can pose risk of infection. The focus of ulcer management is dealing with or preventing infection, reducing foot pressures using offloading devices and an appropriate dressing regime (Williams et al. 2011).

11.11 Management of Nail Conditions

(a) Onychomycosis (OM) is an infection of the nail unit that can be caused by various species of dermatophytes, yeasts, moulds and even some bacteria. OM infects between 2% and 18% of the population with increasing frequency as patient age. With an increases to 20% and 30% for those older than 60 years and 70 years, respectively (Derby et al. 2011), and there is an increased association with immune-compromised patients (Cherry et al. 2017; Bodman et al. 2003). Bodman et al. (2003) also identified that if OM is left untreated, it can lead to subungual and skin ulceration, in patients with RA. Treatment of onychomycosis includes:

- Regular podiatry treatment. Thorough debridement of all dystrophic and hypertrophic nail plates to relieve painful pressure and facilitate topical agent penetration to the nail bed. This also allows the podiatrist to check for subungual ulceration.
- Topical therapy. Topical lacquers such as Trosyl (tioconazole), Loceryl (amorolfine) and Lamisil (terbinafine).
- Systemic antifungal therapy is necessary if there is extensive nail involvement. Oral antifungal therapies, e.g. Sporanox (itraconazole) and Lamisil (terbinafine hydrochloride), are used as they have a broad spectrum of activity and require a short duration of treatment. However, there are many possible contraindications which require caution when prescribing and as such may not be recommended for people with RA or SLE, including:
  - Hepatic and renal impairment
  - Risk of exacerbation of psoriasis
  - Risk of lupus erythematosus-like effect
  - Pregnant and nursing mothers
  - Drug interactions

(b) Onychocryptosis (ingrowing toe nail) is a common problem for which patients seek podiatry treatment. The nail may puncture the soft tissue and allow bacterial invasion resulting in paronychia (inflammation and swelling around the nail) and infection, often accompanied by hypergranulation tissue. Conservative treatment may resolve the issue, and if there is infection then antibiotic therapy is advised. However, persistent infections or acute pain may require that the nail is removed totally or partially under local anaesthetic. Podiatrists are trained in nail surgery and can carry out these procedures following written agreement by the patient's consultant (Fig. 11.5).

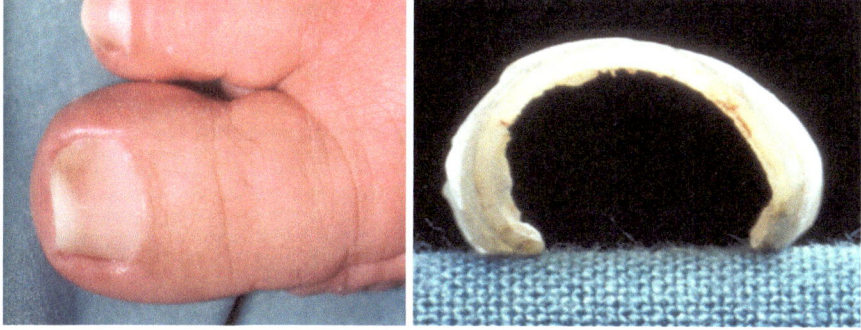

Fig. 11.5 Ingrowing toe nail (onychocryptosis) caused by excessive curvature of the nail plate (total removal of the nail)

11.12 Steroid Injection Therapy

The structures of the foot and ankle in RA and SLE are particularly susceptible to inflammation and are amenable to both diagnostic and therapeutic injection of steroid. This therapy allows for specific targeting of localised joints which may be symptomatic even though the general disease process is controlled by oral medications. Therefore, the main indication for use of therapeutic injection therapy is for active joint inflammation and pain relief but only in the absence of sepsis.

Administering steroids via the intra-articular or localised soft tissue approaches has advantages over oral use of steroids. Typical systemic side effects seen with steroids are reduced and improvement can be rapid. Ward et al. (2008) found improvement following corticosteroid injection up to and including 6 months post injection. Common sites for injection include the ankle joint, subtalar joint, first metatarsophalangeal joint, interphalangeal joints, the plantar fascia, interdigital spaces, the tarsal tunnel, retro-calcaneal bursae and tendon sheaths of the peroneal and posterior tibial tendons.

The benefit gained from injection therapy depends on a number of factors:

- Correct diagnosis of the presenting complaint
- Appropriateness of injection therapy as treatment option
- Degree of inflammation
- Accurate placement of the injection
- Type of steroid used
- The amount of rest following the injection
- Correction of any structural deformity using orthoses

All these factors contribute to both the benefit and duration of benefit from injection therapy. In the foot, accurate placement is sometimes difficult and often injections are guided using X-ray screening or ultrasound (U/S). Without guidance, accuracy of placement depends purely on the skill of the practitioner. Using X-ray guidance often leads to delay in performing the injection and exposes the patient to radiation. U/S guidance is seen as the way forward and is likely to become more common as clinicians are trained in the modality and the technology becomes cheaper and more readily available (Brown et al. 2004). As with any invasive procedure, there are potential risks, which the referring practitioner needs to be aware of and the administering practitioner needs to consider before injection is carried out and discussed with the patient before informed consent is obtained.

There is believed to be a higher risk of post injection infection associated with injections in the foot and ankle. However, anecdotally, this risk is reported to be low if good aseptic techniques are adopted for any joint or soft tissue injection procedure.

11.13 Foot Surgery

Whilst it is recognised that advances in the medical management of RA with biologic therapies has seen a reduction in the requirement for orthopaedic surgery, many patients with the disease will go on to develop problems with their feet and ankles that may require a surgical opinion. People with RA should be referred for an early specialist surgical opinion if any of the following do not respond to optimal non-surgical management:

• Persistent pain due to joint damage or other identifiable soft tissue cause
• Worsening joint function
• Progressive deformity
• Persistent localised synovitis

(NICE guidelines 2009)
Reasons for surgical referral may include:

• Persistent pain, stiffness, synovitis in the foot or ankle joints, tenosynovitis or tendon ruptures, loss of function (Loveday et al. 2012)
• Foot deformities causing restriction in mobility due to pain or recurrent ulceration
• Osteomyelitis/septic arthritis
• It is generally accepted that referrals for surgical opinion should be considered for patients with RA when optimum conservative management has failed to bring their symptoms to an acceptable level. A potential exceptions is early synovectomy in severe disease, to prevent rapid joint destruction (Canseco et al. 2011)

11.14 Summary

Foot problems can be the manifestation of rheumatic diseases in the older person and can impact on mobility, functional ability and stability. Foot problems in people with rheumatic diseases are common and involve the structure and function of the foot, the vascular and neurological supply to the foot and the skin and toe nails. General foot care advice given by nurses can maintain or improve foot health and compliment specialist foot care interventions.

Identification and timely referral of people with pain and inflammation affecting the joints of the feet is important in preventing deterioration of foot structure/function.

Further, identification and urgent referral of people with clinical signs of infection affecting the feet is crucial to prevent infection spreading systemically. Also, identification and urgent referral of people with clinical signs of vascular problems affecting the feet are crucial to prevent loss of tissue viability and ultimately loss of toes. Clearly feet need to be part of a nurse's assessment of the older person to facilitate appropriate advice, timely referral and early intervention in order to minimise the pain, functional limitation and disability caused by foot problems.

11.15 Self-Assessment

Having read the chapter and undertaken further study, the following are some ideas as how to relate what you have learnt to your practice:

1. Consider how you *currently* assess an older person's feet.
2. Reflect on key aspects of foot health that you could introduce into your assessment.
3. What actions can you introduce to ensure that a patient's foot health needs are met?
4. What are the urgent foot problems that need immediate referral? Consider how this could be facilitated to ensure timely intervention.
5. Identify the foot problems that need to be referred for specialist (surgical and podiatry) interventions.
6. Discuss with your colleagues how to deliver basic foot health advice to enable self-care.

References

ARMA. Arthritis and musculoskeletal alliance – standards of care for people with inflammatory arthritis. 2004. Available from: http://www.arma.uk.net.

ARMA Guidelines. Standards of care for people with connective tissue diseases. 2004. Available from: http://www.arma.uk.net/pdfs/ctdweb.pdf. Accessed 11 Jan 2013.

Barn R, Turner DE, Rafferty D, Sturrock RD, Woodburn J. Tibialis posterior tenosynovitis and associated pes plano valgus in rheumatoid arthritis: electromyography, multisegment foot kinematics, and ultrasound features. Arthritis Care Res (Hoboken). 2013;65(4):495–502.

Blake A, Mandy PJ, Stew G. Factors influencing the patient with rheumatoid arthritis in their decision to seek podiatry. Musculoskeletal Care. 2013;11:218.

Bodman MA, Feder L, Nace AM. Topical treatments for onychomycosis: a historical perspective. J Am Podiatr Med Assoc. 2003;93(2):136–41.

Brenton-Rule A, Dalbeth N, Menz HB, Bassett S, Rome K. Foot and ankle characteristics associated with falls in adults with established rheumatoid arthritis: a cross-sectional study. BMC Musculoskelet Disord. 2016;17(1):22.

Brown AK, O'Connor PJ, Wakefield RJ, Roberts TE, Karim Z, Emery P. Practice, training, and assessment among experts performing musculoskeletal ultrasonography: toward the development of an international consensus of educational standards for ultrasonography for rheumatologists. Arthritis Rheum. 2004;51(6):1018–22.

Canseco K, Albert C, Long J, Khazzam M, Marks R, Harris GF. Postoperative foot and ankle kinematics in rheumatoid arthritis. J Exp Clin Med. 2011;3(5):233–8.

Cherry L, Alcacer-Pitarch B, Hopkinson N, Teh LS, Vital EM, Edwards CJ, et al. The prevalence of self-reported lower limb and foot health problems experienced by participants with systemic lupus erythematosus: results of a UK national survey. Lupus. 2017;26:410–6.

Davys HJ, Turner DE, Helliwell PS, Conaghan PG, Emery P, Woodburn J. Debridement of plantar callosities in rheumatoid arthritis: a randomized controlled trial. Rheumatology (Oxford). 2005;44(2):207–10.

Derby R, Rohal P, Jackson C, Beutler A, Olsen C. Novel treatment of onychomycosis using over-the-counter mentholated ointment: a clinical case series. J Am Board Fam Med. 2011;24(1):69–74.

Dixon WG, Watson K, Lunt M, Hyrich KL, Silman AJ, Symmons DP, et al. Rates of serious infection, including site-specific and bacterial intracellular infection, in rheumatoid arthritis patients receiving anti-tumor necrosis factor therapy: results from the British Society for Rheumatology Biologics Register. Arthritis Rheum. 2006;54(8):2368–76.

Emery P, Breedveld FC, Dougados M, Kalden JR, Schiff MH, Smolen JS. Early referral recommendation for newly diagnosed rheumatoid arthritis: evidence based development of a clinical guide. Ann Rheum Dis. 2002;61(4):290–7.

Firth J, Helliwell P, Hale C, Hill J, Nelson EA. The predictors of foot ulceration in patients with rheumatoid arthritis: a preliminary investigation. Clin Rheumatol. 2008;27(11):1423–8.

Göksel Karatepe A, Günaydin R, Adibelli ZH, Kaya T, Duruöz E. Foot deformities in patients with rheumatoid arthritis: the relationship with foot functions. Int J Rheum Dis. 2010;13(2):158–63.

Graham AS, Stephenson J, Williams AE. A survey of people with foot problems related to rheumatoid arthritis and their educational needs. J Foot Ankle Res. 2017;10:12.

Grondal L, Tengstrand B, Nordmark B, Wretenberg P, Stark A. The foot: still the most important reason for walking incapacity in rheumatoid arthritis: distribution of symptomatic joints in 1,000 RA patients. Acta Orthop. 2008;79(2):257–61.

Hooper L, Bowen CJ, Gates L, Culliford DJ, Ball C, Edwards CJ, et al. Prognostic indicators of foot-related disability in patients with rheumatoid arthritis: results of a prospective three-year study. Arthritis Care Res (Hoboken). 2012;64(8):1116–24.

van der Leeden M, Steultjens MP, van Schaardenburg D, Dekker J. Forefoot disease activity in rheumatoid arthritis patients in remission: results of a cohort study. Arthritis Res Ther. 2010;12(1):R3.

Li CY, Imaishi K, Shiba N, Tagawa Y, Maeda T, Matsuo S, et al. Biomechanical evaluation of foot pressure and loading force during gait in rheumatoid arthritic patients with and without foot orthosis. Kurume Med J. 2000;47(3):211–7.

Loveday DT, Jackson GE, Geary NP. The rheumatoid foot and ankle: current evidence. Foot Ankle Surg. 2012;18(2):94–102.

McElhone K, Abbott J, Gray J, Williams A, Teh LS. Patient perspective of systemic lupus erythematosus in relation to health-related quality of life concepts: a qualitative study. Lupus. 2010;19(14):1640–7.

McEntegart A, Capell HA, Creran D, Rumley A, Woodward M, Lowe GD. Cardiovascular risk factors, including thrombotic variables, in a population with rheumatoid arthritis. Rheumatology (Oxford). 2001;40(6):640–4.

Menz HB, Morris ME. Footwear characteristics and foot problems in older people. Gerontology. 2005;51(5):346–51.

Menz HB, Auhl M, Spink MJ. Foot problems as a risk factor for falls in community-dwelling older people: a systematic review and meta-analysis. Maturitas. 2018;118:7–14.

van Netten JJ, Francis A, Morphet A, Fortington LV, Postema K, Williams A. Communication techniques for improved acceptance and adherence with therapeutic footwear. Prosthetics Orthot Int. 2017;41(2):201–4.

NICE. Guidance for the management of rheumatoid arthritis in adults. 2009. Available from: https://www.nice.org.uk/guidance/cg79.

Riente L, Delle Sedie A, Iagnocco A, Filippucci E, Meenagh G, Valesini G, et al. Ultrasound imaging for the rheumatologist. V. Ultrasonography of the ankle and foot. Clin Exp Rheumatol. 2006;24(5):493–8.

Shi K, Tomita T, Hayashida K, Owaki H, Ochi T. Foot deformities in rheumatoid arthritis and relevance of disease severity. J Rheumatol. 2000;27(1):84–9.

Siddle HJ, Hodgson RJ, O'Connor P, Grainger AJ, Redmond AC, Wakefield RJ, et al. Magnetic resonance arthrography of lesser metatarsophalangeal joints in patients with rheumatoid arthritis: relationship to clinical, biomechanical, and radiographic variables. J Rheumatol. 2012a;39(9):1786–91.

Siddle HJ, Firth J, Waxman R, Nelson EA, Helliwell PS. A case series to describe the clinical characteristics of foot ulceration in patients with rheumatoid arthritis. Clin Rheumatol. 2012b;31(3):541–5.

Siddle HJ, Redmond AC, Waxman R, Dagg AR, Alcacer-Pitarch B, Wilkins RA, et al. Debridement of painful forefoot plantar callosities in rheumatoid arthritis: the CARROT randomised controlled trial. Clin Rheumatol. 2013;32(5):567–74.

Turner DE, Woodburn J. Characterising the clinical and biomechanical features of severely deformed feet in rheumatoid arthritis. Gait Posture. 2008;28(4):574–80.

Turner DE, Helliwell PS, Emery P, Woodburn J. The impact of rheumatoid arthritis on foot function in the early stages of disease: a clinical case series. BMC Musculoskelet Disord. 2006;21(7):102.

Turner DE, Helliwell PS, Siegel KL, Woodburn J. Biomechanics of the foot in rheumatoid arthritis: identifying abnormal function and the factors associated with localised disease 'impact'. Clin Biomech (Bristol, Avon). 2008;23(1):93–100.

Ward ST, Williams PL, Purkayastha S. Intra-articular corticosteroid injections in the foot and ankle: a prospective 1-year follow-up investigation. J Foot Ankle Surg. 2008;47(2):138–44.

Wickman AM, Pinzur MS, Kadanoff R, Juknelis D. Health-related quality of life for patients with rheumatoid arthritis foot involvement. Foot Ankle Int. 2004;25(1):19–26.

Williams AE, Graham AS. 'My feet: visible, but ignored ...' a qualitative study of foot care for people with rheumatoid arthritis. Clin Rehabil. 2012;26(10):952–9.

Williams AE, Davies S, Graham A, Dagg A, Longrigg K, Lyons C, et al. Guidelines for the management of the foot health problems associated with rheumatoid arthritis. Musculoskeletal Care. 2011;9(2):86–92.

Williams AE, Crofts G, Teh LS. 'Focus on feet'—the effects of systemic lupus erythematosus: a narrative review of the literature. Lupus. 2013;22(10):1017–23.

Williams AE, Cherry L, Blake A, Alcacer-Pitarch B, Edwards C, Hopkinson N, et al. An investigation into the scale and impact of self-reported foot problems associated with systemic lupus erythematosus: a study protocol and survey questionnaire development. Musculoskeletal Care. 2016;14(2):110–5.

Woodburn J, Helliwell PS. Foot problems in rheumatology. Br J Rheumatol. 1997;36(9):932–4.

Woodburn J, Barker S, Helliwell PS. A randomized controlled trial of foot orthoses in rheumatoid arthritis. J Rheumatol. 2002;29(7):1377–83.

Woodburn J, Hennessy K, Steultjens MP, McInnes IB, Turner DE. Looking through the 'window of opportunity': is there a new paradigm of podiatry care on the horizon in early rheumatoid arthritis? J Foot Ankle Res. 2010;3:8.

Further Reading

Frowen P, O'Donnell M, Gordon Burrow J. Neale's disorders of the foot. 8th ed. London: Churchill Livingstone; 2010. ISBN: 9780702030291.

Helliwell PS, Backhouse MR, Siddle HJ. The foot and ankle in rheumatology. 1st ed. Oxford: Oxford University Press; 2019. ISBN: 9780198734451.

Menz H. Foot problems in older people – assessment and management. 1st ed. London: Churchill Livingstone; 2008. ISBN: 9780080450322.

Rome K, McNair P. Management of chronic conditions in the foot and lower leg. 1st ed. London: Churchill Livingstone; 2014. ISBN: 9780702047695.

Self-Management

12

Gretl A. McHugh

12.1 Learning Outcomes

- To develop an awareness and understanding of the importance of self-management in chronic conditions such as arthritis and other rheumatological conditions
- To improve knowledge of techniques/tools and programmes and to support patients with self-management

12.2 Introduction

People with chronic or long-term conditions, such as arthritis and other rheumatological conditions, have to make decisions everyday about their health condition. Self-management is important for those with a chronic condition as these individuals are the ones who are responsible for their daily care over the duration of the disease (Lorig and Holman 2003). Most of the time, people self-manage their condition without seeking health professionals' input through, for example, keeping active, healthy eating and taking prescribed medication. People with chronic conditions may also seek out activities which will make them feel better, for example, belonging to a reading club or volunteering. Self-management often involves actions where individuals are finding their way through health and social care services and taking an active part in their treatment planning with health and social care professionals (Boger et al. 2015). Evidence has shown that patients being involved in their own care and being motivated to manage their chronic condition result in better disease outcomes (Lorig et al. 1999; Wagner et al. 2005).

G. A. McHugh (✉)
School of Healthcare, University of Leeds, Leeds, UK
e-mail: G.A.McHugh@leeds.ac.uk

© Springer Nature Switzerland AG 2020
S. Ryan (ed.), *Nursing Older People with Arthritis and other Rheumatological Conditions*, Perspectives in Nursing Management and Care for Older Adults,
https://doi.org/10.1007/978-3-030-18012-6_12

Often people with chronic conditions need support for self-management from others, such as health professionals, and having this support helps people to develop the knowledge, confidence and skills in order to manage their condition better. The Health Foundation (2015) promotes self-management support in order to manage not only the physical impact of a chronic condition but also the emotional and social impact. Individuals with a rheumatological condition, such as osteoarthritis (OA), are not only affected by physical symptoms, such as pain (discussed in Chapter 7), but the emotional and social impact of living with the condition (discussed in Chapter 8). Having OA often has a profound effect on an individuals' quality of life (Cook et al. 2007; McHugh et al. 2012). There is also evidence of social isolation due to individuals with OA experiencing chronic pain and disability (Smith et al. 2014). Therefore, support and guidance are important for individuals to manage more effectively their symptoms, and of particular value is guided support which is targeted at the individual and the chronic condition.

There is a drive by health governments to ensure that individuals are empowered to shape and manage their own health and make informed choices about their care. It is estimated that around 70–80% of people with a long-term condition (LTC) can be supported to manage their own condition (Department of Health 2005a). The Health Foundation recognises that self-management support is an important component of person-centred care through: 'supporting people to recognise and develop their own strengths and abilities to enable them to live an independent and fulfilling life' (The Health Foundation 2015, p. 6).

Managing a chronic condition is challenging for the older person. Nurses and other health professionals are key to supporting individuals with chronic conditions, such as arthritis, to become more active in managing their own condition more effectively. Evidence from a Department of Health study found that more than 90% of those surveyed were interested in being more active self-carers; and 75% said if they had more guidance from a professional or peer, they would feel more confident in taking care of their own health (Department of Health 2005b).

12.3   Defining Self-Management

Self-management encompasses the skills, confidence and knowledge which the individual needs to develop to manage living with the chronic condition. Self-management is defined as the:

> Day-to-day tasks an individual must undertake to control or reduce the impact of disease on physical health status. At-home management tasks and strategies are undertaken with the collaboration and guidance of the individual's physician and other health care providers. (Clark et al. 1991, p. 5)

Self-care and self-management are often terms used interchangeably. However, self-care is distinguished from self-management in that self-care is considered more as promoting and preventing disease and includes activities performed by healthy individuals at home to maintain health and well-being (Clark et al. 1991; World Health Organization 2014; Department of Health 2009).

Table 12.1 Self-management skills

Self-management skills (Lorig and Holman 2003)	Interpretation
Problem solving	Defining what the problem is and possible solutions for achieving the desired outcome
Decision-making	Having the correct and right amount of information to make an informed decision
Resource utilisation	Teaching people to use resources; how to access and choose from the resources/information available
Formation of patient-provider relationship	Helping to develop partnerships with health professionals
Development of an action plan	Learning how to change behaviour, make an action plan and accomplish the goal/activity. Having the confidence to achieve this
Self-tailoring	Distinguishes self-management from, for example, health promotion. It needs to take into account a person's stage of change or health beliefs

Source: Lorig and Holman (2003)

Self-management involves much more than taking prescribed treatments for the chronic condition; it also includes the emotional, social and psychological management of adjusting to living with the condition and managing the emotional changes which may occur (Barlow et al. 2002). The individual's ability to cope and manage all the feelings and the effects which having the condition brings upon the individual and often the family members is part of the self-management process.

Lorig and Holman (2003) discuss six self-management skills and further interpretation of each provided in Table 12.1.

Self-management shifts the individual with the chronic condition away from passively receiving treatment to empowering the individual to become pro-active in managing their own condition (De Silva 2011). It is important that patients have the self-management skills in order to actively manage and live with their chronic condition.

Self-management tasks which are seen to be common to patients with arthritis include adapting to work, managing the emotional and psychological responses to the condition, using relaxation and stress-reducing techniques, taking medication, maintaining a healthy diet and engaging in exercise (Clark et al. 1991). Across other chronic conditions, such as asthma, diabetes, chronic obstructive pulmonary disease and heart disease, there are commonalities with some of these self-management tasks (Clark et al. 1991).

12.4   Self-Management Support

Having support for self-management from health professionals or others, such as a family member or a peer, is helpful for individuals with chronic diseases. The Institute of Medicine (2003) defines self-management support as:

The systematic provision of education and supportive interventions to increase patients' skills and confidence in managing their health problems, including regular assessment of progress and problems, goal setting, and problem-solving support. (IOM (Institute of Medicine) 2003, p. 52)

The help which is provided to individuals with a chronic condition enables them to manage their health better on a day-to-day basis (Agency for Healthcare Research and Quality 2019). Self-management support is not just about the health professional giving information to the patient, but it is helping them to learn about their condition, set goals and make plans for a healthier life. It encourages a partnership and therefore a better relationship between the patient and health professional.

Both the health professional and the patient with the chronic condition have responsibilities for managing the condition. It is important that patients are active partners in determining what goals are important to them and how these could be achieved, through working in partnership with healthcare professionals (The Health Foundation 2015). For example, the patient might want to increase their physical activity but doesn't really know how to do the most effective exercises. By working in collaboration with the health professional and being supported, the patient will be better placed to achieve their goal of increasing physical activity.

Kennedy et al. (2013) discuss two core models of self-management support: patient-based models, an example of this is the Expert Patient Programme (discussed in Section 12.5), and provider-based models, which include embedding self-management support within health professionals' consultations (Kennedy et al. 2014; CentreForum Mental Health Commission 2014). Kennedy et al. (2013) argue that it is important to embed self-management support within health professionals' consultations, and this makes it more sustainable and accessible by all. However, a patient-based model requires people to attend the programme, and often some programs may be poorly attended or else not attended by those who may benefit.

Areas which are important to consider alongside self-management support are patients having access to the support required, patients having an understanding of person-centred care and self-efficacy and how patients, families and professionals' attitudes can influence engagement with self-management. These topics are briefly discussed in Sections 12.4.1–12.4.6.

12.4.1 Access to Support

It is also essential that the patient is able to access the support they need which might include other organisations than those provided by the health service (The Health Foundation 2015). There are many third-sector organisations, such as Versus Arthritis and Age UK, which help and support individuals with specific condition issues but also provide other support and activities for a healthier life.

Social prescribing is a community-centred approach providing a: 'mechanism for linking patients with non-medical sources of support within the community' (CentreForum Mental Health Commission 2014, p. 6). Social prescribing is recognised as one of a number of community-centred approaches for health and well-being and is seen as a model for providing access to community resources by connecting people to resources, information and social activities, encouraging participation (Public Health England 2015). Sources of support may include, but are not limited to, exercise or art on prescription, creative classes, physical activity, support for housing, gaining employment, self-care and self-help groups, social or luncheon clubs and engaging individuals with volunteer opportunities. A review of community referral schemes has found benefits of social prescribing to include: increases in self-esteem and confidence, a sense of control and empowerment, improvements in psychological well-being and positive mood (Thomson et al. 2015).

There are existing schemes which may assist people with chronic condition in reducing social isolation. In addition, there are a number of specific charities where information and support are available, such as Versus Arthritis. This charity is also training professionals to become 'Musculoskeletal (MSK) Champions' to improve MSK healthcare. In Northern Ireland, there was a befriending programme delivered by volunteers, 'Staying Connected', and a preliminary evaluation provides evidence of its value (McHugh et al. 2018). Similar to volunteers are peer mentors, who are individuals who have the chronic condition and with training, to support and guide individuals with the same condition to self-manage, and this has been found to be an effective approach (Fisher et al. 2017).

12.4.2 Person-Centred Care

Person-centred care is ensuring that individuals are at the forefront of their healthcare. This enables individuals to be in control, helps them share in the decision-making process and supports better partnership working between individuals and their health and social care providers (National Voices 2017). One core component of person-centred care is supporting self-management. Individuals can self-manage independently or in partnership with their healthcare providers. There is often more cooperation with self-management when there is encouragement to self-manage by health professionals.

12.4.3 Self-Efficacy

Self-efficacy is important in self-management, in terms of one's ability to cope with the chronic condition. Self-efficacy is defined by Bandura as an individual's ability to succeed in specific situations or tasks (Bandura 1977). Having the confidence to achieve goals/tasks is important. The level of confidence is important for the individual to believe that he/she is capable of actually accomplishing the activities/goals set. If a person lacks self-efficacy, individuals do not manage situations effectively despite having the required skills and ability (Bandura 1990).

12.4.4 Patient Engagement

Engagement is a vital element for self-management, and the individual has responsibilities to engage in activities that promote health. For example, in osteoarthritis, exercise is important (NICE 2014), and the individual, once guided and instructed in the optimal exercises, must try and engage with this. Engagement with information to support self-management has been an issue. A review found that giving written information increased knowledge, but the evidence that this helped informed choice was poor (Fox 2006). Information needs to be specific and targeted for the chronic condition. A qualitative review found that how information is provided and by whom and when information is given are important aspects to consider and successful for patient engagement and therefore more effective in supporting self-management (Protheroe et al. 2008).

Patients will vary considerably in their engagement and participation in self-management. A patient's commitment to a treatment or to an intervention will often depend on their willingness to make changes in their behaviours, for example, starting to exercise or adjusting their diet. This willingness to change may depend on an individual's stage of change which include (Prochaska and DiClemente 1983):

- Pre-contemplation: where the individual has no intention of changing behaviour.
- Contemplative: the individual is aware of the problem, but no commitment to change.
- Preparation: individual is ready to change.
- Action: individual is actively changing/modifying behaviour.
- Maintenance: change occurs.

'Relapse', that is, falling back to old ways/habit, is an integral component of the stages of change and needs to be considered. The stages of change (described above) are one component of the 'transtheoretical model of behaviour change' which also incorporates the process of change and ways to measure change (Prochaska and DiClemente 1983).

A study to understand the adoption of arthritis self-management identified groups based on the transtheoretical model of stages of change (Prochaska and DiClemente 1983): precontemplation, contemplation, preparation, unprepared action and prepared maintenance. The study, concluded by tailoring treatment to the patients' state of change, may enhance the outcomes of self-management interventions for arthritis (Keefe et al. 2000).

It is also important to identify the potential barriers that patients may have in engagement with self-management support opportunities. A US study explored barriers to accessing self-management support resources for chronic conditions and found that there was often a lack of awareness, physical symptoms, transport problems and insurance to cover finances which prevented individuals from accessing available help (Jerant et al. 2005).

12.4.5 Family Engagement

Families are key in supporting self-management. A review found that families needed knowledge about the chronic condition including how best to support management, in particular coping with the emotional issues which individuals with a chronic condition may experience (Boger et al. 2015).

12.4.6 Professional Engagement

Professional engagement to support self-management is also key. There have been difficulties in embedding and implementing self-management in healthcare. One study found that if patients don't take responsibility for their health, often this affects the motivation of nurses to engage with and support self-management activities (Kennedy et al. 2014). A European study found that even though nurses were self-confident in their ability to support self-management, there were barriers such as the nurses' time but also the patients' lack of knowledge (Van Hooft et al. 2016). A study explored the barriers to general practitioners referring patients with osteoarthritis to self-management programmes and found that a lack of knowledge and a negative attitude to these programmes were key referral barriers (Pitt et al. 2008).

It is also important to understand the roles, responsibilities and relationships between individuals with chronic conditions and the health and social care professionals who support them (The Health Foundation 2015). The health practitioner needs to incorporate skills in self-management in order to optimise their consultations with patients. Building up a relationship with the patient is important, and ensuring the use of good communication skills (see Section 12.5.5) and techniques, such as motivational interviewing (see Section 12.5.3), is essential.

Putting in place systems, procedures and training for healthcare professionals may help with embedding self-management support in their interaction with patients with chronic conditions (The Health Foundation 2015). However, with other health priorities within primary care, the work required to implement self-management support is difficult within the current systems and often is not given priority to becoming an integral part of primary care consultations (Kennedy et al. 2014). There are many challenges to implementing self-management into current healthcare systems and as part of health professionals' work (Lorig and Holman 2003). One study looked at an enhanced general practitioner consultation to improve self-management of osteoarthritis using a 'Whole Systems Informing Self-Management Engagement (WISE) model' for guided self-management (Kennedy et al. 2013), and although some improvements were shown from the clinical trial, the main outcome of an improvement in physical functioning at 6 months was not evident (Dziedzic et al. 2018).

Ensuring that all health professionals have a common understanding on how best to support patients with self-management, including the engagement with the appropriate self-management tools and techniques, is of value. Reminders to health professionals in organisations as to what support may be available to patients with chronic conditions, such as peer support interventions, self-management programmes, befriending organisations and social prescribing, would be of value and would assist the health professional in their consultations with patients.

12.5   Self-Management Tools and Techniques

There are many techniques and tools to help patients develop and maintain healthy behaviours. The main ones which will be discussed are action planning and goal setting, patient activation, motivational interviewing, health coaching and communication.

12.5.1 Action Planning and Goal Setting

Developing an action plan is important to co-produce with patients. There are several ways to develop an action plan. Figure 12.1 provides an example of an individual with knee osteoarthritis, who would like to lose weight. Weight management is important in the management of osteoarthritis (NICE 2014). When developing an action plan with the patient, it is necessary to set the goals to achieve the activity. Having clear goals are important for achieving high quality of care (Dixon-Woods et al. 2014). Goal setting is a vital component of self-management. Goals set by the individual with a chronic condition needs to be carefully thought about. Goals should be specific, measurable, achievable, realistic and time-bound, summarised in the mnemonic 'SMART' (Doran 1981) and now used widely in healthcare (Bovend'Eerdt et al. 2009). The setting of specific goals and evaluating progress are key to successful self-management. Discussed in Chapter 7, the use of SMART goals is recommended and can be helpful in health professionals' consultations in

Fig. 12.1 Example of an action plan using SMART goals

Action Plan

Goal: To lose weight

SMART GOAL:
Specific: To lose 7 pounds
Measurable: To lose ½ to 1 pound per week
Achievable (or appropriate): Level of importance between 1–10: 9
Realistic: Level of confidence of achieving between 1–10: 6
Time bound: To lose 7 pounds in 2 months

Barriers to achieving goal: Family celebrations coming up

Plans to overcome barriers: Choose lower calorie food at the family celebration events

Evaluation measure: Will keep a weekly progress of weight loss

working with the patient to ensure activities are directed towards achieving the best outcome. When setting SMART goals, if the level of importance set by the patient is less than 7 (out of 10), then the patient may have to set another goal which has higher importance for them. The goal must be realistic, and this covers the level of confidence in achieving the goal, and if the patient scores less than 7 for this component, the health professional needs to assess how this confidence level could be increased. Often confidence can be increased through discussing with the patient their previous experience of change: what has helped and what strategies were used to change the behaviour for this situation, as this may be beneficial for other situations. It may be necessary to re-assess the level of confidence. It might also be helpful to discuss any barriers to achieving the goal, for example, what is getting in the way of achieving their desired weight loss and discuss ways to overcome the barrier (Fig. 12.1).

Similar to action planning is agenda setting and is an approach which enables the patient to set their own agenda in the session with the health practitioner. The patient is in control, and it encourages both the patient and the practitioner to work towards goals. Often used are 'importance/confidence measures', and these are ruler scales where the patient would mark how important change is to them and how confident they feel that they can achieve the goal. This enables the practitioner to see how motivated the patient is to change and assess the level of confidence. Often the barriers to achieving progress are brought out, and these can be discussed with the patient to find out what the obstacles might be to achieving change.

12.5.2 Patient Activation

To measure and understand more about engagement with a person's own health and health behaviours, NHS England promotes the use of a 'Patient Activation Measure' (PAM®), a tool which is a short questionnaire that health professionals or organisations use to understand a patient's activation levels, that is, the knowledge, skills and confidence an individual has in order to manage his/her chronic condition (NHS England 2019a; Hibbard and Gilburt 2014). There are specific questions which the patient completes, for example, about his/her knowledge of prescribed medication or on how to prevent problems with his/her health. Some health organisations are using PAM® to understand the 'activation level' of their patients and therefore modify their services for more individualised person-centred care. If patients are measured at the lower levels of activation (levels 1 and 2), individuals are unlikely to engage and may be overwhelmed with the opportunities to improve self-management of their chronic condition, whereas if measured at the higher levels (3 and 4), patients are taking action and are building or establishing self-management skills. Using a tool such as the PAM® questionnaire enables the health professional or organisation to have a clearer understanding of where and at what level the patient is at so as to tailor their support and if appropriate deliver the right intervention to improve and increase patient activation.

12.5.3 Motivational Interviewing

Motivation, listening and coaching are all tools which can support self-management and help individuals to make changes. In order to help individuals to change their behaviour and identify their problems and do something about it, motivational interviewing (MI) is recommended as an approach when working with patients/individuals with health issues. MI was developed in part by Rollnick and Miller (1995) and is defined as a: 'skillful clinical style for eliciting from patients their own good motivations for making behavior changes in the interest of their own health' (Miller and Rollnick 1991, p. 6).

MI involves a semi-directive approach that enables health professionals to question and support patients. Health professionals can use open-ended questions and provide positive affirmation, showing an understanding with what the patient is saying as well as reflecting upon what is being said. There are principles which the health professional become trained to adhere to, and a brief description of these principles are provided in Table 12.2.

Motivational interviewing has been found to be helpful in the treatment of rheumatoid arthritis (RA), through helping to increase medication adherence and physical activity and improve coping strategies for symptoms of pain and fatigue which patients with RA experience (Georgopoulou et al. 2016).

Motivational interviewing can help people to change their behaviours with the health professional helping patients to understand their feelings towards changing their behaviour. It is important to identify any of the barriers to change and look at what the individuals' strengths are. It will enable individuals to feel in control of their decisions and help achieve a person-centred approach to care. The health professional is key to using motivational interviewing successfully in their consultations with patients.

12.5.4 Health Coaching

Health coaching uses techniques of motivational interviewing. Health coaching is seen to increase patients' activation and motivation to self-manage (Lindner et al.

Table 12.2 Principles of motivational interviewing

Principles	Description
Express empathy	Being attentive and listening to the patient; being empathetic; acknowledging what the patient has said and putting it in your own words as the health professional
Roll with resistance	Recognising resistance; helping the patient move away from the perceived obstacles and barriers
Support self-efficacy	Recognising the change which has been successful previously and support the patient to achieve change; build on their motivation
Develop discrepancy	Helping the patient see how their behaviour may stop them from achieving his/her goal

Source: Rollnick and Allison (2004, pp.109–110)

2003). Trained health coaches support individuals to set a goal, for example, walking to the shop. The health coach will work with patient to achieve this goal by breaking this activity down into more manageable steps, for example, a first step might be initially walking to the front gate, and then the next steps may include gradually increasing the distance over a number of weeks until the goal is achieved. Health coaching may involve the use of the PAM questionnaire (see Section 12.5.2) to assess how prepared the patient is and the level of confidence the patient has. From a review of the evidence, health coaching helps in the management of chronic conditions (The Evidence Centre and Health Education East of England 2014).

12.5.5 Communication

Communication between the patient and health professional is very important and can be challenging for individuals with a chronic condition. Evidence has found that many individuals with chronic diseases encounter issues with communicating with a health professional which can be difficult and distressing to them (Thorne et al. 2000).

Specifically, in individuals with osteoarthritis, there can be discordance between the patient and doctor, and this was evident when the general practitioner normalised the symptoms of OA as part of life (Paskins et al. 2015). A narrative review found that patients wanted doctors to acknowledge symptoms and provide specialist knowledge and education which was personalised for the patient (Paskins et al. 2014).

At times there may be different goals between the health professional and patient. The health professional may be more interested in the management of the condition, whereas the patient is more focused on the ability to take part in activities which are important to them. At times, there is a mismatch of goals between the patient and the health professional (Heisler et al. 2003). There may be differing expectations regarding the outcome of the consultation between the patient and the health professional; and at times there may need to be a process of negotiation and reshaping of these expectations. It is important during a consultation that the health professional clarifies the patient's expectation of the consultation at the beginning; as when there is better alignment between the needs of the patient with the health professional, this achieves better engagement and results. Good communication between the patient and health professionals is important in managing a chronic condition effectively.

12.6 Self-Management Interventions

There are a number of self-management programmes and interventions which have been developed to help individuals manage their chronic condition. These are delivered in different formats and include being delivered by lay or professional people: those which are disease specific, e.g. arthritis focused, or generic specific, e.g. for chronic conditions, and those which are group or individually delivered (Barlow et al. 2002; Coster and Norman 2009). Self-management programmes often focus on patient-perceived problems, and these types of programmes tend to be effective in improving behaviours and self-efficacy (Lorig and Holman 2003).

A review of the evidence to support self-management found that different types of interventions, such as self-management education, using electronic technology, self-monitoring and training health professionals in self-manage-ment support, are beneficial in improving: knowledge, patient experience, ser-vice use and costs, health behaviours and outcomes (National Voices 2014). However, the evidence and outcomes vary depending on type of chronic condi-tion. For example, programs which teach self-management skills show more improvement in outcomes than information only interventions (Bodenheimer et al. 2002).

Providing patients with education to encourage self-management is common. After receiving self-management education, short-term improvements in health sta-tus were found, but these were not always sustained in the long term (Niedermann et al. 2004; Warsi et al. 2003; Du et al. 2011).

Specifically, for arthritis, a review of self-management interventions found that the main focus was to reduce pain and improve physical and psychological functioning (Newman et al. 2004). The key characteristics of the interventions tended to be where much of the responsibility is taken by the individual with the chronic condition (Newman et al. 2004). This review found that in around 40% of self-management interventions for arthritis, there was an improvement in self-reported symptoms and measures of disability (Newman et al. 2004). Although the long-term sustained effects on pain and disability are questionable.

One of the earliest arthritis self-management programmes showed improve-ments in pain and depression and a reduction in health service use (Lorig and Holman 2003; Lorig et al. 1985). Another self-management programme in pri-mary care specifically for patients with arthritis, which consisted of six sessions of self-management with an educational booklet found that there was a reduc-tion in anxiety and an improvement in perceived self-efficacy, but there was no significant effect on pain, physical function or primary care consultations (Buszewicz et al. 2006). When data from this study and eight other studies on self-management programmes for individuals with osteoarthritis were com-bined using meta-analyses, self-management interventions had limited clinical benefit in terms of pain, function and depression and in reducing health profes-sional consultations, but there was evidence of improved knowledge (Smith et al. 2013).

There are other self-management programmes which are specific to managing chronic pain referred to as pain management programmes; and there is evidence to support the effectiveness of these programmes (Gauntlett-Gilbert and Brook 2018; Morley et al. 2013).

A generic programme known as the Stanford Chronic Disease Self-Management Programme (CDSMP) has been in existence since the late 1990s and has undergone further development (Lorig et al. 1999, 2001). This programme is grounded in self-efficacy (discussed in Section 12.4.3). This self-management programme provides six structured sessions delivered by lay leaders with a focus on collaborative goal setting, personalised problem solving and developing skills and knowledge (Brady et al. 2013; Battersby et al. 2007). Studies have shown improvements in self-efficacy, health behaviours and health status, with less hospital visits (Lorig et al. 1999, 2001). A meta-analysis of studies of outcomes from the CDSMP showed that there were small to moderate improvements in psychological health and other health behaviours that were still evident after 12 months of completing the CDSMP (Brady et al. 2013). Other well-known generic programmes are the Flinders Chronic Care Management Programme, which focuses more on the patient defining the goals and not the health professional (Battersby et al. 2007; Lawn and Schoo 2010).

In the UK, the Expert Patient Programme (EPP) developed in 2001 is a 6 week lay-led delivered programme available to individuals who identify themselves as having a chronic condition (Newbould et al. 2006; Rogers 2019). Evaluations of the EPP revealed an increase in self-efficacy, but no reduction in the use of health services (Rogers 2019; Kennedy et al. 2007).

A review of the evidence of lay-led self-management found benefits but also problems associated with these programmes (Newbould et al. 2006). However, there is evidence to suggest that the generic self-management courses delivered by lay-people are less effective than disease specific self-management education where professionals are involved as part of routine healthcare (Kennedy et al. 2014; National Voices 2014).

Another programme which is supported by the NHS specifically for chronic arthritic pain is the ESCAPE-Pain (Enabling Self-management and Coping with Arthritic Pain through Exercise) programme (NHS England 2019b). Approved by the National Institute for Health and Care Excellence (NICE) as a rehabilitation programme, this programme was initially developed as a face-to-face programme, and there is strong evidence to support its effectiveness (Hurley et al. 2007, 2012).

With so many advances in technology with the use of telehealth, which include helplines, the Internet and mobile phone apps, there are other formats to deliver self-management interventions and programmes. An Internet-based arthritis self-management programme was found to be effective at improving health status and was seen as a feasible alternative to a face-to-face group arthritis self-management programme (Lorig et al. 2008). The ESCAPE-Pain programme is now available digitally, so individuals can have access to the right exercise programmes to manage their chronic hip or knee pain (NHS Innovation Accelerator 2018).

The self-management programmes and interventions discussed in this section are just a few of the many programmes and initiatives available to help support and teach individuals to acquire the skills and knowledge and help build the confidence to manage their chronic condition.

In summary, with our ageing population, increasing number of individuals with arthritis and other rheumatological conditions and the current strain on our health and social care providers, there is a need for effective self-management by individuals with chronic conditions. Nurses and other health professionals must play an active role in supporting and helping patients to achieve effective self-management.

Summary of Main Points
1. Self-management is important for individuals living with a chronic condition such as arthritis.
2. Engagement with self-management is necessary by patient, families and health professionals.
3. Goal setting is a key component for effective self-management.
4. Motivational interviewing is a technique which helps guides the patient to make a decision about behaviour change.
5. Good communication between the patient and health professional is necessary and important for developing a partnership.
6. Self-management programmes and interventions can be effective in teaching the individual skills and knowledge and building confidence to manage a chronic condition.

12.7   Self-Assessment (Suggested Further Study)

1. Consider and discuss what self-management support you could offer an older person who has arthritis.
2. Think of a goal to be addressed with a patient who has arthritis; complete the SMART approach to goal setting in Table 12.3.

Table 12.3 SMART approach

SMART	Patient's issue
Specific goal	
Measurable goal	
Achievable goal	
Realistic goal	
Time-bound	

3. For an individual who is not confident in achieving a goal in relation to self-management of arthritis, discuss ways in which you could support the patient to be more confident.
4. Discuss ways in which you could encourage a better partnership between patients and a health professional.

References

Agency for Healthcare Research and Quality. Self management support—content last reviewed October 2018. 2019. http://www.ahrq.gov/professionals/prevention-chronic-care/improve/self-mgmt/index.html. Accessed 19 Jan 2019.

Bandura A. Self-efficacy: toward a unifying theory of behavioural change. Psychol Rev. 1977;84(2):191–215. https://doi.org/10.1037/0033-295X.84.2.191.

Bandura A. Perceived self-efficacy in the exercise of control over AIDS infection. Eval Prog Policy. 1990;13:9–17.

Barlow J, Wright C, Sheasby J, Turner A, Hainsworth J. Self-management approaches for people with chronic conditions: a review. Patient Educ Couns. 2002;48:177–87.

Battersby M, Harvey P, Mills PD, Kalucy E, Pols RG, Firth PA, et al. SA HealthPlus: a controlled trial of a statewide application of a generic model of chronic illness care. Millbank Q. 2007;85:37–67. https://doi.org/10.1111/j.1468-0009.2007.00476.x.

Bodenheimer T, Lorig K, Holman H, Grumbach. Patient self-management of chronic disease in primary care. JAMA. 2002;288(19):2469–75.

Boger E, Ellis J, Latter S, Foster C, Kennedy A, Jones F, et al. Self-management and self-management support outcomes: a systematic review and mixed research synthesis of stakeholder views. PLoS One. 2015;10(7):1–25. https://doi.org/10.1371/journal.pone.0130990.

Bovend'Eerdt TJH, Botell RC, Wade DT. Writing SMART rehabilitation goals and achieving goal attainment scaling: a practical guide. Clin Rehabil. 2009;23:352–61. https://doi.org/10.1177/0269215508101741.

Brady TJ, Murphy L, O'Colmain BJ, Beauchesne D, Daniels B, Greenberg M, et al. A meta-analysis of health status, health behaviors, and health care utilisation outcomes of the chronic disease self-management program. Prev Chronic Dis. 2013;10:1–14. https://doi.org/10.5888/pcd10.120112.

Buszewicz M, Rait G, Griffin M, Nazareth I, Patel A, Atkinson A, et al. Self management of arthritis in primary care: randomized controlled trial. BMJ. 2006;333:879. https://doi.org/10.1136/bmj.38965.375718.80.

CentreForum Mental Health Commission. The pursuit of happiness: a new ambition for our mental health. London: CentreForum; 2014.

Clark NM, Becker MH, Janz NK, Lorig K, Rakowski W, Anderson L. Self-management of chronic disease in older adults: a review and questions for research. J Ageing Health. 1991;3(1):3–27. https://doi.org/10.1177/089826439100300101.

Cook C, Pietrobon R, Hegedus E. Osteoarthritis and the impact of quality of life health indicators. Rheumatol Int. 2007;27:315–21. https://doi.org/10.1007/s00296-006-0269-2.

Coster S, Norman I. Cochrane reviews of educational and self-management interventions to guide nursing practice: a review. Int J Nurs Stud. 2009;46(4):508–28. https://doi.org/10.1016/j.ijnurstu.2008.09.009.

De Silva D. Evidence: helping people help themselves. A review of the evidence considering whether it is worthwhile to support self-management. London: The Health Foundation; 2011.

Department of Health. Supporting people with long-term conditions: an NHS and social care model to support local innovation and integration. London: Department of Health; 2005a.

Department of Health. MORI survey: public attitudes to self care baseline survey. London: Department of Health; 2005b.

Department of Health. Your health your way – a guide to long term conditions and self care. London: Department of Health; 2009.

Dixon-Woods M, Baker R, Charles K, Dawson J, Jerzembek G, Martin G, et al. Culture and behavior in the English National Health Service: overview of lessons from a large multimethod study. BMJ Qual Saf. 2014;23(2):106–15. https://doi.org/10.1136/bmjqs-2013-001947.

Doran GT. There's a S.M.A.R.T way to write management's goal and objectives. Manag Rev. 1981;70(11):35–6.

Du S, Yuan C, Xiao X, Chu J, Qiu Y, Qian H. Self-management programs for chronic musculoskeletal pain conditions: a systematic review and meta-analysis. Patient Educ Couns. 2011;85(3):e299–310. https://doi.org/10.1016/j.pec.2011.02.021.

Dziedzic KS, Healey EL, Porcheret M, Afolabi EK, Lewis M, Morden A, et al. Implementing core NICE guidelines for osteoarthritis in primary care with a model consultations (MOSAICS): a cluster randomised controlled trial. Osteoarthr Cartil. 2018;26:43–53. https://doi.org/10.1016/j.joca.2017.09.010.

Fisher EB, Boothroyd RI, Elstad EA, Hays L, Henes A, Maslow GP, et al. Peer support of complex health behaviors in prevention and disease management with special reference to diabetes: systematic reviews. Clin Diabetes Endocrinol. 2017;3(4) https://doi.org/10.1186/s40842-017-0042-3.

Fox R. Informed choice in screening programmes: do leaflets help? A critical literature review. J Public Health (Oxf). 2006;28(4):309–17.

Gauntlett-Gilbert J, Brook P. Living well with chronic pain: the role of pain-management programmes. BJA Educ. 2018;18(1):3–7. https://doi.org/10.1016/j.bjae.2017.09.001.

Georgopoulou S, Pothero L, Lempp H, Galloway J, Sturt J. Motivational interviewing: relevance in the treatment of rheumatoid arthritis? Rheumatology (Oxford). 2016;55:1348–56. https://doi.org/10.1093/rheumatology/kev379.

Heisler M, Vijan S, Anderson RM, Ubel PA, Bernstein SJ, Hofer TP. When do patients and their physicians agree on diabetes treatment goals and strategies, and what difference does it make? J Gen Intern Med. 2003;18(11):893–902.

Hibbard J, Gilburt H. Supporting people to manage their health: an introduction to patient activation. The King's Fund. 2014. www.kingsfund.org.uk/sites/default/files/field/field_publication_file/supporting-people-manage-health-patient-activation-may14.pdf. Accessed 16 Jan 2019.

Hurley MV, Walsh NE, Mitchell HL, Pimm TJ, Patel A, Williamson E, et al. Clinical effectiveness of a rehabilitation program integrating exercise, self-management, and active coping strategies for chronic knee pain: a cluster randomized trial. Arthritis Rheum. 2007;57(7):1211–9. https://doi.org/10.1002/art.22995.

Hurley MV, Walshe NE, Mitchell H, Nicholas J, Patel A. Long-term outcomes and costs of an integrated rehabilitation program for chronic knee pain: a pragmatic, cluster randomized, controlled trial. Arthritis Care Res. 2012;64(2):238–47. https://doi.org/10.1002/acr.20642.

IOM (Institute of Medicine). In: Adams K, Corrigan JM, editors. Priority areas for national action: transforming health care quality. Washington, DC: National Academy Press; 2003.

Jerant AF, von Friederichs-Fitzwater MM, Moore M. Patients' perceived barriers to active self-management of chronic conditions. Patient Educ Couns. 2005;57:300–7. https://doi.org/10.1016/j.pec.2004.08.004.

Keefe FJ, Lefebvre JC, Kerns RD, Rosenberg R, Beaupre P, Prochaska J, et al. Understanding the adoption of arthritis self-management: stages of change profiles among arthritis patients. Pain. 2000;87:303–13.

Kennedy A, Reeves D, Bower P, Lee V, Middleton E, Richardson G, et al. The effectiveness and cost effectiveness of a national lay-led self care support programme for patients with long-term conditions: a pragmatic randomised controlled trial. J Epidemiol Community Health. 2007;61(3):254–61. https://doi.org/10.1136/jech.2006.053538.

Kennedy A, Bower P, Reeves D, Blakeman T, Bowen R, Chew-Graham C, et al. Implementation of self-management support for long term conditions in routine primary care settings: cluster randomised controlled trial. Br Med J. 2013;346:f2882. https://doi.org/10.1136/bmj.f2882.

Kennedy A, Rogers A, Bowen R, Lee V, Blakeman T, Gardner C, et al. Implementing, embedding and integrating self-management support tools for people with long-term conditions in primary care nursing: a qualitative study. Int J Nurs Stud. 2014;51:1103–13. https://doi.org/10.1016/j.ijnurstu.2013.11.008.

Lawn S, Schoo A. Supporting self-management of chronic health conditions: common approaches. Patient Educ Couns. 2010;80:205–11. https://doi.org/10.1016/j.ppec.2009.10.006.

Lindner H, Menzies D, Kelly J, Taylor S, Shearer M. Coaching for behavior change in chronic disease: a review of the literature and the implications for coaching as a self-management intervention. Aust J Prim Health. 2003;9:177–85.

Lorig KR, Holman HR. Self-management education: history, definition, outcomes and mechanisms. Ann Behav Med. 2003;26(1):1–7. https://doi.org/10.1207/S15324796ABM2601_01.

Lorig K, Lubeck D, Kraines RG, Seleznick M, Holman HR. Outcomes of self-help education for patients with arthritis. Arthritis Rheum. 1985;28:680–5.

Lorig KR, Sobel DS, Stewart AL, Brown BW Jr, Bandura A, Ritter P, et al. Evidence suggesting that a chronic disease self-management program can improve health status while reducing hospitalization: a randomized trial. Med Care. 1999;37:5–14.

Lorig KR, Ritter P, Steward AL, Sobel DS, Brown BW Jr, Bandura A, et al. Chronic disease self-management program: 2-year health status and healthcare utilization outcomes. Med Care. 2001;39:1217–23.

Lorig KR, Ritter PL, Laurent DD, Plant K. The internet-based arthritis self-management programme: a one-year randomized trial for patients with arthritis or fibromyalgia. Arthritis Care Res. 2008;59(7):1009–17. https://doi.org/10.1002/art.23817.

McHugh GA, Campbell M, Luker KA. Quality of care in individuals with osteoarthritis: a longitudinal study. J Eval Clin Pract. 2012;18(3):534–41. https://doi.org/10.1111/j.1365-2753.2010.01616.x.

McHugh GA, Conaghan PG, McConville M, Cullen A, Hadi MA, Kingsbury SR. Promoting self-management in older people with arthritis: preliminary findings of the Northern Ireland Staying Connected Programme. Musculoskeletal Care. 2018;16:489–93. https://doi.org/10.1002/msc.1353.

Miller WR, Rollnick S. Motivational interviewing: preparing people to change addictive behavior. New York: Guilford Press; 1991.

Morley S, Williams A, Eccleston C. Examining the evidence about psychological treatments for chronic pain: time for a paradigm shift? Pain. 2013;154:1929–31.

National Voices. Supporting self-management. 2014. https://www.nationalvoices.org.uk/sites/default/files/public/publications/supporting_self-management.pdf. Accessed 11 Jan 2019.

National Voices. Person-centred care in 2017. London: National Voices; 2017.

Newbould J, Taylor D, Bury M. Lay-led self-management in chronic illness: a review of the evidence. Chronic Illn. 2006;2:249–61. https://doi.org/10.1177/17423953060020040401.

Newman S, Steed L, Mulligan. Self-management interventions for chronic illness. Lancet. 2004;364:1523–37. https://doi.org/10.1016/S0140-6736(04)17277-2.

NHS England. Patient activation. 2019a. https://www.england.nhs.uk/ourwork/patient-participation/self-care/patient-activation/. Accessed 16 Jan 2019.

NHS England. NHS long term plan. 2019b. Available from: https://www.longtermplan.nhs.uk. Accessed 5 Feb 2019.

NHS Innovation Accelerator. Award-winning ESCAPE-pain programme now online. 2018. https://nhsaccelerator.com/award-winning-escape-pain-programme-now-online/. Accessed 5 Feb 2019.

NICE. Osteoarthritis: care and management. 2014. https://www.nice.org.uk/guidance/cg177. Accessed 19 Jan 2019.

Niedermann K, Fransen J, Knols R, Uebelhart D. Gap between short-and long-term effects of patient education in rheumatoid arthritis patients: a systematic review. Arthritis Rheum. 2004;51(3):388–98. https://doi.org/10.1002/art.20399.

Paskins Z, Sanders T, Hassell AB. Comparison of patient experiences of the osteoarthritis consultation with GP attitudes and beliefs to OA: a narrative review. BMC Fam Pract. 2014;15:46. https://doi.org/10.1186/1471-2296-15-46.

Paskins Z, Sanders T, Croft PR, Hassell AB. The identity crisis of osteoarthritis in general practice: a qualitative study using video-stimulated. Ann Fam Med. 2015;13(6):537–44. https://doi.org/10.1370/afm.1866.

Pitt VJ, O'Connor D, Green S. Referral of people with osteoarthritis to self-management programmes: barriers and enablers identified by general practitioners. Disabil Rehabil. 2008;30(25):1938–46. https://doi.org/10.1080/09638280701774233.

Prochaska JO, DiClemente CC. Stages and processes of self-change of smoking: toward an integrative model of change. J Consult Clin Psychol. 1983;51:390–5.

Protheroe J, Rogers A, Kennedy AP, Macdonald W, Lee V. Promoting patient engagement with self-management support information: a qualitative meta-synthesis of processes influencing uptake. Implement Sci. 2008;3:44. https://doi.org/10.1186/1748-5908-3-44.

Public Health England. A guide to community-centred approaches for health & wellbeing. London: Public Health England & NHS England; 2015.

Rogers A. Expert patients' programme: evidence expert review – NICE. 2019. https://www.nice.org.uk/guidance/ph19/evidence/expert-paper-1-pdf-371292301. Accessed 6 Feb 2019.

Rollnick S, Allison J. Motivational interviewing. In: Heather N, Stockwell T, editors. The essential handbook of treatment and prevention of alcohol problems. Hoboken, NJ: Wiley; 2004. p. 105–16.

Rollnick S, Miller WR. What is motivational interviewing? Behav Cognit Psychother. 1995;23:325–34.

Smith TO, Davies L, McConnell L, Cross J, Hing CB. Self-management programmes for people with osteoarthritis: a systematic review and meta-analysis. Curr Rheumatol Rev. 2013;9:165–75.

Smith TO, Purdy R, Lister S, Salter C, Fleetcroft R, Conaghan P. Living with osteoarthritis: a systematic review and meta-ethnography. Scan J Rheumatol. 2014;43(6):441–52. https://doi.org/10.3109/03009742.2014.894569.

The Evidence Centre and Health Education East of England. Does health coaching work? Summary of key themes from a rapid review of empirical evidence. The Evidence Centre and Health Education East of England. 2014. https://eoeleadership.hee.nhs.uk/sites/default/files/Does%20health%20coaching%20work%20-%20a%20review%20of%20empirical%20evidence_0.pdf. Accessed 13 Jan 2019.

The Health Foundation. A practical guide to self-management support. Key components for successful implementation. London: The Health Foundation; 2015.

Thomson LJ, Camic PM, Chatterjee HJ. Social prescribing: a review of community referral schemes. London: UCL; 2015.

Thorne SE, Ternulf Nyhlin K, Paterson BL. Attitudes toward patient expertise in chronic illness. Int J Nurs Stud. 2000;37:303–11.

Van Hooft SM, Dwarswaard J, Bal R, Strating MM, van Staff AL. What factors influence nurses' behavior in supporting patient self-management? An explorative questionnaire study. Int J Nurs Med. 2016;63:65–72. https://doi.org/10.1016/j-ijnurstu.2016.08.017.

Wagner EH, Bennett SM, Austin BT, Greene SM, Schaefer JK, Vonkorff M. Finding common ground: patient-centeredness and evidence-based chronic illness care. J Altern Complement Med. 2005;11(Suppl 1):s7–s15. https://doi.org/10.1089/acm.2005.11.s-7.

Warsi A, LaValley MP, Wang PS, Avorn J, Solomon DH. Arthritis self-management education programs: a meta-analysis of the effect on pain and disability. Arthritis Rheum. 2003;48(8):2207–13. https://doi.org/10.1002/art.11210.

World Health Organization. Regional Office for South-East Asia. Self care for health. WHO Regional Office for South-East Asia. 2014. http://www.who.int/iris/handle/10665/205887. Accessed 15 Jan 2019.

Further Reading

Carrier J. Managing long-term conditions and chronic illness in primary care. A guide to good practice. Oxford: Routledge; 2015. ISBN: 978-0415-65717-4.

Lorig K, Holman H, Sobel D, Laurent D, González V, Minor M. Self-management of long-term health conditions. A handbook for people with chronic disease. Boulder, CO: Bull Publishing Company; 2014. ISBN: 978-1936693627.

National Voices. Supporting self-management. 2014. https://www.nationalvoices.org.uk/sites/default/files/public/publications/supporting_self-management.pdf. Accessed 19 Aug 2019.